Anshan Gold Standard Mini Atlas Series

Oral Medicine

System requirement:
- **Windows XP or above**
- **Power DVD player (Software)**
- **Windows media player 10.0 version or above (Software)**

Accompanying CD Rom is playable only in Computer and not in CD player.

Kindly wait for few seconds for CD to autorun. If it does not autorun then please follow the steps:
- Click on my computer
- Click the **CD drive labelled JAYPEE** and after opening the drive, kindly double click the file **Jaypee**

Anshan Gold Standard Mini Atlas Series

Oral Medicine

Anil Ghom BDS, MDS
Professor and Head
Department of Oral Medicine and Radiology
Chhattisgarh Dental College and Research Center
Sundra, Rajandagao, Chhattisgarh
India

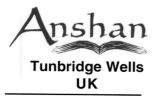

**Tunbridge Wells
UK**

JAYPEE BROTHERS
MEDICAL PUBLISHERS (P) LTD.
New Delhi

First published in the UK by

Anshan Ltd
in 2008
6 Newlands Road
Tunbridge Wells
Kent TN4 9AT, UK

Tel: +44 (0)1892 557767
Fax: +44 (0)1892 530358
E-mail: info@anshan.co.uk
www.anshan.co.uk

ISBN 13   978-1-905740-38-3

British Library Cataloguing in Publication Data
A catalogue record for this book is available from the British Library

Printed in India by Ajanta Offset & Packagings Ltd., New Delhi

Many of the designations used by manufacturers and sellers to distinguish their
products are claimed as trademarks. Where those designations appear in this book
and where the publisher was aware of a trademark claim, the designations have
been printed in initial capital letters.

This book is dedicated
in the loving memory of my father
late Govindrao W Ghom and
my brother-in-law Late Manish Lodam

This book
radiologist
spinal
a large num
that dentist
clinical
This
best to p
radiographic
I wish this book
can't some answers

Preface

People may doubt what you say
But they will always believe what you do

This book seeks to assist dental students, dentists and radiologists to make informed clinical decision on the optimal management of patient. This atlas is designed with a large number of clinical and radiological photographs so that dentists, students and physicians are able to have clinical and theoretical knowledge of oral disease.

This atlas comprises of 23 chapters and I tried my level best to provide high quality clinical photographs and radiographs in this book.

I wish this book may help the students of dentistry to learn some diseases.

Anil Ghom
Sanvil@rediffmail.com
anil_ghom@yahoomail.com

Contents

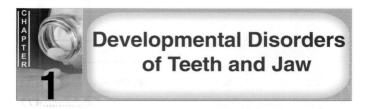

Developmental Disorders of Teeth and Jaw

DEVELOPMENTAL DISTURBANCES OF THE JAWS

Agnathia

It is also called as *'hypognathous'*. It is a extremely rare congenital defect characterized by absence of maxilla or mandible. There may be absent ears, absent or hypoplastic tongue, cleft palate, dysplastic ears, hypertelorism, microstomia and narrow auditory canal.

Micrognathia

It means small jaws and either maxilla or mandible may be affected. It can be apparent (It is due to abnormal positioning or abnormal relation of one jaw to another, which produces illusion of Micrognathia) or true (it is due to small jaw). It can be congenital or acquired in origin. In many instances it is associated with other *congenital abnormalities*, particularly congenital heart disease and Pierre-Robin syndrome (cleft palate, micrognathia, glossoptosis). Acquired type is postnatal type and result from disturbances in the area of *temporomadibular joint* (Ankylosis) (Fig. 1.1).

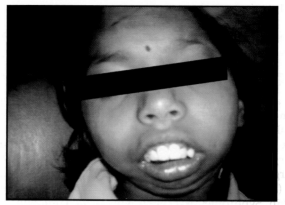

Fig. 1.1: Acquired type of micrognathia of mandible
seen in patient of ankylosis

Clinically it is the one of the cause of abnormal alignment of teeth. This can be seen by observing the occlusion of teeth. In true micrognathia, the jaw is small enough to interfere with feeding of the infant and may require special nipples in order to feed adequately.

It is managed by surgical and orthodontic treatment.

Macrognathia

It refers to the condition of abnormally large jaws. It is also called as *'megagnathia'*. It is hereditary in nature. Some other causes are *pituitary gigantism, Paget's disease of bone, acromegaly and leontiasis ossea.*

Mandibular protrusion or proganthism is common.

There is much "show" when the patient smiles, so that there is a so-called "gummy" smile. This is due to the upper jaw being too long. There is prominent chin button.

It is managed by osteotomy.

Facial Hemihypertrophy

It is also called as *'Friedreich's disease'*. It is caused by hormonal imbalance, incomplete twinning and chromosomal abnormalities.

It may occur alone or in generalized hemihypertrophy. Enlargement of one half of the head present since birth. Enlarged side grows at a rate proportional to uninvolved side (Fig. 1.2). Pigmentation and hemangioma may occur on skin. Syndromes associated with facial hemihypertrophy

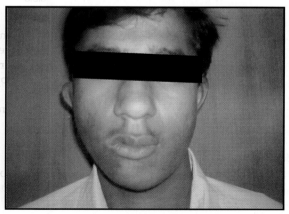

Fig. 1.2: Facial hemihypertrophy on left side the patient

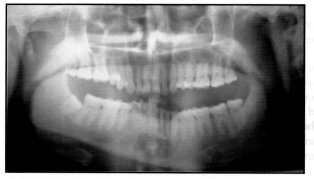

Fig. 1.3: Facial hemihypertrophy seen on left side (*Courtesy*: Dr Datarkar, Asso. Professor, Oral and Maxillofacial Surgery, SPDC, Wardha, India)

are Proteus syndrome and Klippel-Trenaunay-Weber syndrome. Rate of development of permanent teeth on the affected side is more rapid and erupt before their counter-parts on the uninvolved side.

Radiologically enlargement of bone on affected area. The malar bone, zygomatic process and temporal bone may be enlarged in all diameter (Fig. 1.3). The alveolar process is enlarged in some cases.

It is managed by cosmetic repair.

Facial Hemiatrophy

It is also called as *'Parry-Romberg syndrome'*. It is a rare disorder characterized by slowly progressive wasting (atrophy) of the soft tissues of half of the face (hemifacial atrophy).

It is caused by atrophic malfunction of cervical sympathetic nervous system, trauma, infection and hereditary factors.

Onset noted as a white line furrow or mark on one side of face or brow near midline. In rare cases, the disorder is apparent at birth. Severe headache, visual abnormalities, nausea and vomiting occurs. There is graying (blanching) of hair. Many individuals also experience atrophy of half of the upper lip and tongue. There is reduced growth of jaws and eruption of teeth is retarded. There is also malocclusion on the affected side.

Radiologically reduction in size of bone on affected side. Reduction in size of condyle, coronoid process or overall dimension of body and ramus of mandible. The affected side of the face is smaller in all dimensions than the opposite side (Fig. 1.4).

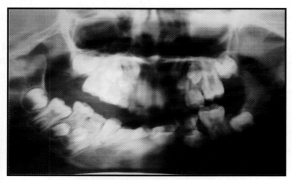

Fig. 1.4: Notice reduced jaw size on left side as compared to on right side

It is managed by orthodontic treatment, plastic surgery and hearing aids.

Cleidocranial Dysplasia

It is also called as *'cleidocranial dysostosis'*, *'Marie and sainton disease'*, *'craniocleido-dysostosis'*.

It is hereditary and when inherited, it appears as a true dominant Mendelian characteristic.

It primarily affects skull, clavicle and dentition. There may be complete absence of clavicle and patients have unusual mobility being able to bring their shoulders forward until they meet in midline (Fig. 1.5). The head is brachycephalic (reduced anterior-posterior dimension but increased skull width) or wide and short. Nasal bridge is depressed with a broad base.

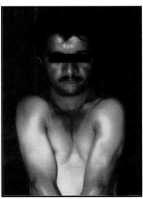

Fig. 1.5: Unusual mobility of shoulders results in due to absence of clavicle

Maxilla and paranasal sinus are underdeveloped, resulting in maxillary micrognathia. Prolonged retention of primary dentition and delayed eruption of permanent dentition. Numerous unerupted teeth are found which are most prevalent in the mandibular premolar and incisor area (Fig. 1.6). There is presence of supernumerary teeth usually in anterior region.

Radiologically skull film reveals open sutures, presence of wormian bones, widened cranium, delayed ossification of fontanelles, frontal and occipital bossing and basilar invagination. Examination of chest reveals malformation and absence of clavicles (Fig. 1.8). Jaw examination reveals prolonged retention of primary dentition, multiple supernumerary teeth and small under-developed jaw (Fig. 1.7).

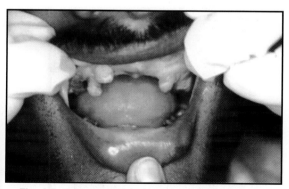

Fig. 1.6: Enamel hypoplasia and delayed eruption of teeth seen in patient of cleidocranial dysplasia

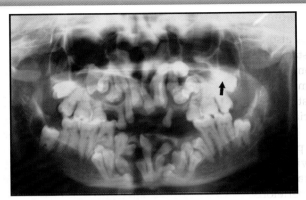

Fig. 1.7: Radiographs showing multiple supernumerary tooth and retention of primary dentition

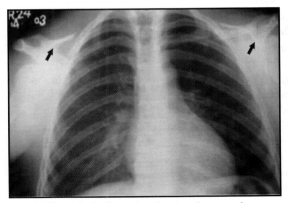

Fig. 1.8: Radiographs showing absence of clavicle in cleidocranial dysostosis

Craniofacial Dysostosis

It is also called as *'Crouzon's disease or syndrome'*. In some instances, Crouzon syndrome is inherited as an autosomal dominant trait. In other cases, affected individuals have no family history of disease. The disorder is characterized by distinctive malformations of the skull and facial (craniofacial) region.

Facial abnormalities typically include unusual bulging or protrusion of the eyeballs (proptosis) due to shallow eye cavities. Outward deviation of one of the eyes (divergent strabismus or exotropia); widely spaced eyes (ocular hypertelorism). There is protuberant frontal region with an anterior-posterior ridge overhanging the frontal eminence and often passing to the root of nose (triangular frontal defect).

Maxillary hypoplasia with shortened antero-posterior dimension of maxillary arch. Dental arch width is reduced and this gives an appearance of highly arch palate (Fig. 1.10). In some cases, facial angle is exaggerated and the patient nose is prominent and pointed, resembling 'parrot beak'. Unilateral or bilateral cross-bite is evident (Fig. 1.9).

Radiologically digital marking in skull as a result of increased intracranial pressure from early synostosis of cranial sutures. The cranial walls are thin with multiple radiolucencies appearing as depressions or scalloped appearance of 'beaten silver' (Fig. 1.11).

Maxillofacial surgery for correction of facial deformities.

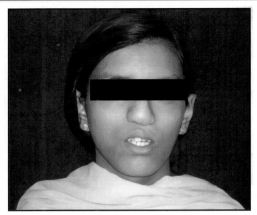

Fig. 1.9: Patient is having Crouzon's syndrome. Note parrot beak and bulging of frontal bone in midline

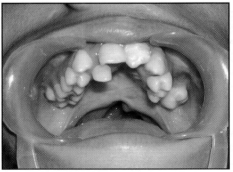

Fig. 1.10: High arch with cross bite in patient with Crouzon's syndrome

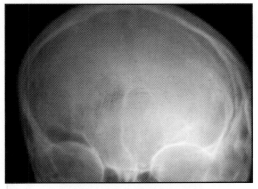

Fig. 1.11: Skull feautres shows beaten silver appearance
(not typical) in Crouzon's syndrome

Mandibulofacial Dysostosis

It is also called as *'Treacher-Collin syndrome'* and *'Franceschetti syndrome'*.

Underdevelopment of zygomatic bone, results in midfacial deformities. Craniofacial malformations includes underdeveloped (hypoplastic) or absent cheek (malar) bone. Downward inclination of palpebral fissure. There is deficiency of eyelashes. There is varying degree of visual impairment in some cases. Affected infants may also have underdeveloped (Fig. 1.12) (hypoplastic) and/or malformed (dysplastic) ears (pinnae) with blind ending or absent external ear canals (microtia), resulting in hearing impairment (conductive hearing loss). Absence of external auditory canal resulting in partial or complete deafness.

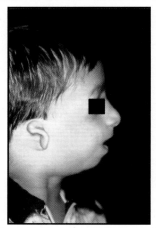

Fig. 1.12: Patient of Treacher-Collins
syndrome showing malformed ear

Underdevelopment of mandible with steep mandi-bular angle. Facial appearance sometimes resembles fish or bird (Fig. 1.13). High arch palate with cleft palate.

Radiologically there is reduction in size of zygomatic bone. Maxillary sinus is underdeveloped or completely absent (Fig. 1.14). Articular eminence is either shallow or absent. Hypoplasia of mandible and maxilla showing accentuation of antegonial notch and steep mandibular angle, which gives impression that the mandible is bending in an inferior and posterior direction (Fig. 1.15).

Cosmetic improvement and surgical interventions to improve osseous and ear defect.

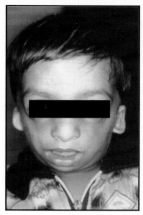

Fig. 1.13: Patient showing bird face appearance
in Treacher-Collins syndrome

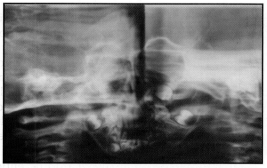

Fig. 1.14: Underdeveloped maxillary sinus in case of
Treacher-Collins syndrome

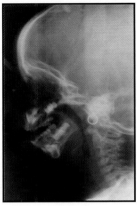

Fig. 1.15: Hypoplasia of mandible showing impression that mandible is bending in inferior and posterior direction

Phlebectasia

This term is first used by Gerwig in 1928. It is an isolated, abnormal, fusiform or saccular dilatation of veins. It is also known as *venous congenital cyst, venous aneurysm, venous ectasia or essen-tial venous dilatation.*

It is caused by mechanical compression of left innominate vein by a high tortuous aorta in hypertension or of venous structures between the sternum and the left innominate artery in pectus excavatum.

Usually appears as isolated swelling. Swelling is not visible before the compression (Fig. 1.16) but as soon as patient clinch the jaws swelling is visible (Fig. 1.17).

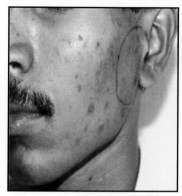

Fig. 1.16: Without compression of neck no swelling is visible

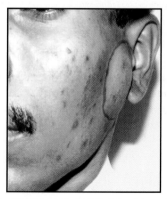

Fig. 1.17: Note the swelling seen on left side of face below the ear after the compression (*Courtesy*: Dr Abhishek Soni, Lecturer, Periodontia, VSPM Dental College and Research Center, Nagpur, India)

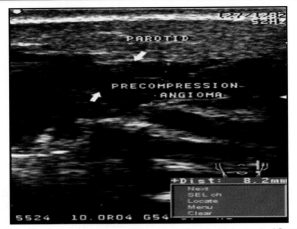

Fig. 1.18: Decompression image on sonography of phlebectasia (*Courtesy*: Dr Abhishek Soni, Lecturer, Periodontia, VSPM Dental College and Research Center, Nagpur, India)

Ultrasonography—dilated blood vessels are usually seen on ultrasonography (Fig. 1.18).

Venography—dilated venous channels seen on venography (Fig. 1.19).

It is managed by surgical, embolisation or injection of sclerosing agents.

Gardner Syndrome

It is also called as familial multiple polyposis. It is hereditary conditions.

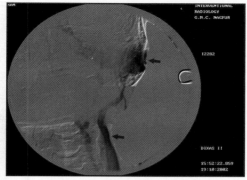

Fig. 1.19: Venography picture of jugular vein, venous dilatation (green arrow) and left jugular vein (red arrow) (*Courtesy*: Dr Abhishek Soni, Lecturer, periodontia, VSPM Dental College and Research Center, Nagpur, India)

Osteomas (Fig. 1.20) are most common in frontal bone, mandible, maxilla and sphenoid bone. There is presence of unerupted supernumerary teeth (Fig. 1.21) in the jaws. There may be cutaneous sebaceous cyst, subcutaneous fibroma, and multiple polyp or small and large intestine.

DEVELOPMENTAL DISTURBANCES OF SIZE OF TEETH

Microdontia

It refers to teeth that are smaller than normal.

Peg shaped lateral is the one of the common form of localized microdontia in which the mesial and distal sides converges or taper incisally, forming peg shaped or cone shaped crown (Fig. 1.22).

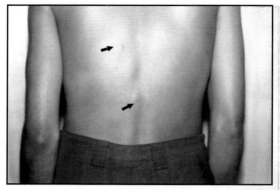

Fig. 1.20: Osteoma seen on back of patient (*Courtesy*: Dr Datarkar, Asso. Professor, Department of Oral Surgery, SPDC, Wardha, India)

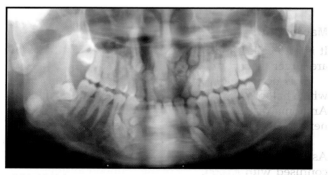

Fig. 1.21: Multiple supernumerary teeth seen in case of Gardner syndrome (*Courtesy*: Dr Datarkar, Asso. Professor, Department of Oral Surgery, SPDC, Wardha, India)

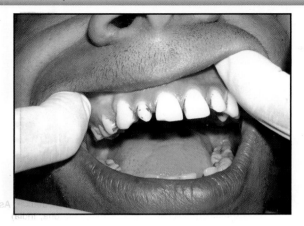

Fig. 1.22: Peg shaped right lateral incisor

Macrodontia

It is also called as *'megadontia'*. These are the teeth which are larger than normal (Fig. 1.23).

It is occasionally seen in facial hemi-hypertrophy, in which half of the teeth in unilateral distribution are affected. Angioma of face, pituitary gigantism and genetic component.

There is crowding, which may result in malocclusion. As space is less, there is impaction of teeth. It should not be confused with fusion.

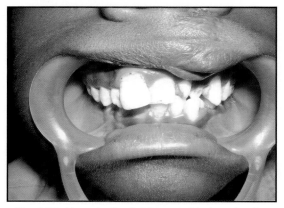

Fig. 1.23: Macrodontia of right central incisor showing large size as compare to adjacent tooth

SHAPE OF TEETH

Gemination

It refers to the process whereby, single tooth germ invaginates resulting in incomplete formation of two teeth that may appear as bifid crown on single root. It occurs during the proliferation stage of the growth cycle of tooth.

It appears clinically as bifid crown on single root.

Fusion

It is also called as *'synodontia'*. It represents the embryonic union of normally separated tooth germs. It represents junction at the level of dentin between juxtaposed normal tooth germs. It can be complete or incomplete (Fig. 1.24).

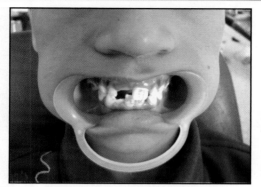

Fig. 1.24: Fusion left lateral incisor and left central incisor

It is transmitted as autosomal dominant trait with reduced penetration. Physical force or pressure generated during development causes contact of tooth germs.

It may occur between a normal tooth and a supernumerary tooth such as *'mesiodens'* or *'distomolar'*. Tooth is almost twice in size than normal, with or without bifid crown. Tooth may have separate or fused root canals (Fig. 1.25). Dental caries is common in fused teeth.

Endodontic treatment should be carried out.

Concrescence

It is a form of fusion that occurs after the root and other major parts involved in teeth are formed or when the roots of two or more teeth are united by cementum, below the cementoenamel junction. It is also called as *'false gemination'*. It can be congenital or acquired.

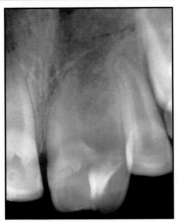

Fig. 1.25: Fusion of teeth with confluent dentin (*Courtesy*: Dr Amit Parate, Lecturer, Oral Medicine and Radiology, GDCH, Nagpur, India)

It is caused by traumatic injury, overcrowding of the teeth with resorption and interdental bone loss.

It usually involved are only two teeth, roots are fused by cementum (Fig. 1.26). Teeth may fail to erupt or incompletely erupt. There may be malocclusion or the teeth may be impacted.

Diagnosis is made by radiographs. Dentist must be careful while doing extraction.

Talon's Cusp

It projects lingually from cingulum area of maxillary and mandibular teeth or it is an anomalous hyperplasia of

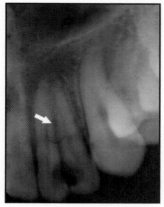

Fig. 1.26: Fusion tooth by roots (*Courtesy:* Dr Mody, Professor and Head, Oral Medicine and Radiology, GDCH, Nagpur, India)

cingulum on the lingual of maxillary and mandibular incisors, resulting in the formation of supernumerary cusp.

It resembles like an *'Eagle's talon'*. It blends smoothly with the erupted tooth, (Fig. 1.27) except that there is deep a developmental groove where the cusp blends with sloping lingual tooth surface. Cusp may or may not contain pulp horn and is usually 'T' shaped. It is associated with Rubinstein-Taybi syndrome.

Radiologically outline is smooth and a layer of normal appearing enamel is distinguishable.

Removal of cusp followed by endodontic therapy.

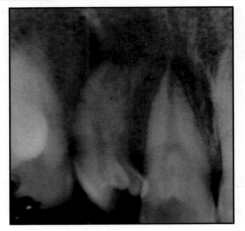

Fig. 1.27: Talon cusp seen as projected radiopacity

Dilaceration

It refers to angulations or sharp bends or curve in the roots and crowns of the teeth (Fig. 1.28). It is cause by mechanical trauma, developmental defect.

There is curve or bending occurs anywhere along the length of tooth, sometimes at cervical portion or midway along the root or even just at the apex of root. Sometimes, angles are so acute that a tooth does not erupt.

Radiologically it will show angular distortion of unusual relationship between coronal and radicular portion of the tooth, on either side of defect (Fig. 1.28).

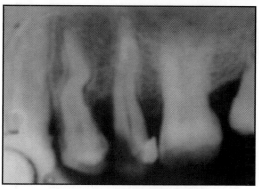

Fig. 1.28: Dilaceration of root in a very unusual way (*Courtesy*: Dr Mody, Professor and Head, Oral Medicine and Radiology, GDCH, Nagpur, India GDCH, Nagpur, India)

Dens in Dente

It is also called as *'dens invaginatus'* or *'dilated composite odontome'* or *'gestant odontome'*. Infolding of the outer surface of the tooth into its interior surface occurs (Fig. 1.29). It is a developmental variation which is thought to arise as a result of an invagination in the surface of crown before calcification.

It can be *coronal dens invaginatus* or *radicular dens invaginatus*.

In coronal type there is a deep pit in cingulum (mild), pocket of enamel is formed within tooth (moderate), it may exhibit an invagination extending nearly to the apex of the root (severe). In some cases there appears to be a grossly

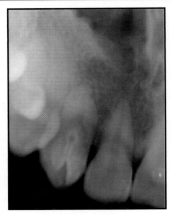

Fig. 1.29: Infolding seen as greater
radiodensity in lateral incisor

magnified cingulum rising to the level of the incisive edge
of the tooth, but lacking the normal contour of a cingulum.

In radicular type crown is small, short and conical with
small orifice at the extreme summit of the convexity. Lingual
marginal ridge is prominent.

Radiologically infolding is recognized by its greater
radiodensity (Fig. 1.29). In radicular type it appears as a
poorly defined, slightly radiolucent structure running
longitudinally within the root. The tooth resembles *'inverted
open umbrella'*, the handle of which is short, being represented
by the conical, nipple-shaped crown.

Tooth should be treated prophylactically.

Dens Evaginatus

It is also called as *'Leong's premolar'*, *'evaginated odontome'* or *'occlusal enamel pearl'*. Dens evaginatus is a developmental condition that appears clinically as an accessory cusp or globules of enamel on occlusal surface, between buccal and lingual cusps of premolar.

Radiologically dentin core is covered with opaque enamel. Fine pulp horns may be apparent.

If tubercle is a cause of occlusal interference, it should be removed under aseptic conditions.

Taurodontism

It is described in 1913 by *Sir Arthur Keith*. In this, body of tooth is enlarged at the expense of root. It is characterized by clinical and anatomical crown of normal shape and size, an elongated body and short roots with longitudinally enlarged pulp chambers.

It is cause by failure of Hertwig's epithelial root sheath to invaginate at proper horizontal level.

It can be hypotaurodont, mesotaurodont and hypertaurodont.

Involved teeth tend to be of rectangular shape rather than the normal tapering towards root (Fig. 1.30). In hypertaurodont, the bifurcation or trifurcation occurs near the apex of root. It is associated with Klinefelter syndrome and Trichodentoosseous syndrome.

Radiologically pulp chamber is extremely large with much greater apicoocclusal height than normal (Fig. 1.30). Extensions of rectangular pulp chamber into elongated body of the tooth.

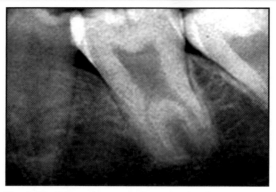

Fig. 1.30: Enlarged, rectangular pulp chamber extending in to the elongated body of the tooth

Supernumerary Roots

Teeth that are normally single rooted exhibit two roots. They develop as slender outgrowths at the center of furcation area of molar teeth (Fig. 1.31).

Radiologically if the two apices are on the labial and lingual side they may get superimposed on each other appearing as a bulbous root, which may mimic hyper-cementosis.

NUMBER OF TEETH

Anodontia

It is congenital absence of teeth. It is caused by hereditary ectodermal dysplasia, cleidocranial dysplasia, craniofacial

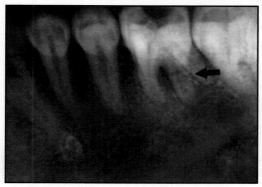

Fig. 1.31: Supernumerary root (red arrow)
seen in relation with first molar

dysostosis and cleft lip and palate, genetic factors,
evolutionary trend towards few teeth and X-ray radiation
(Fig. 1.32).

It can be total (oligodontia) or partial (hypodontia). In
partial anodontia there is absence of one or more teeth.
Commonly missing are 3rd molar, maxillary lateral incisor,
maxillary or mandibular 2nd premolar.

Ectodermal Dysplasia

It is also called as *'hereditary hypohidrotic (anhidrotic)
ectodermal dysplasia'*. It is a X-linked, recessive mendelian
character.

It is characterized by hypotrichosis, hypohidrosis and
anhidrosis with saddle nose appearance. The hair of scalp
and eyebrows tend to be fine, scanty and blond (Fig. 1.33).

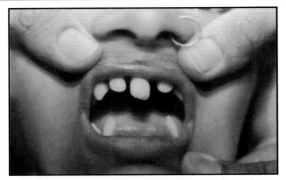

Fig. 1.32: Hypodontia showing missing central incisor on left side

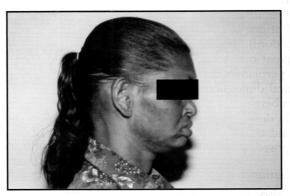

Fig. 1.33: Hereditary ectodermal dysplasia showing
dry skin and sparse hair on the scalp

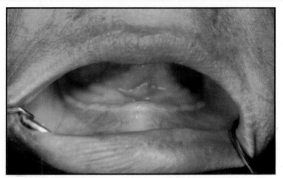

Fig. 1.34: Ectodermal dysplasia showing absence of teeth

Supraorbital and frontal bosses are pronounced. Skin is often dry, soft, smooth and scaly with partial or complete absence of sweat glands.

Patient with this abnormality invariably manifest oligodontia (Fig. 1.34) or partial absence of teeth, with frequent malformation of any present tooth in deciduous and permanent dentition. There is reduction of the normal vertical dimension of alveolar ridge (Fig. 1.35) resulting in protuberant lips.

In dental point of view partial and complete dentures should be constructed for both functional and cosmetic purpose.

Supernumerary Teeth

It is also called as 'hyperdontia'. It is associated with cleft palate, cleidocranial dysplasia, orofacial digital syndrome and Gardner's syndrome.

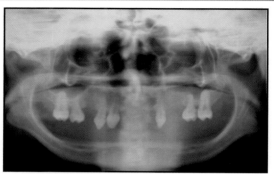

Fig. 1.35: Ectodermal dysplasia showing absence of teeth and thin alveolar ridge

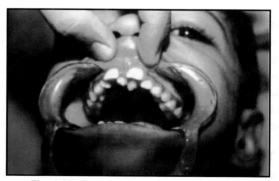

Fig. 1.36: Supernumerary teeth seen in upper anterior region in central incisor area

It can be mesiodense (in the midline in the incisal (Fig. 1.36) region of maxilla between central incisors) distomolar

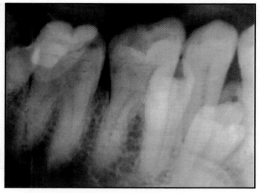

Fig. 1.37: Supernumerary impacted tooth seen molar area

(found in molar region frequently located distal to 3rd molar) Para molar (situated buccally or lingually to one of the maxillary molars or inter-proximally between 1st, 2nd and 3rd maxillary molars) and peridens (Fig. 1.37) (erupt ectopically, either buccally or lingually to the normal arch are referred as peridens). Occlusal radiograph will aid in deter-mining the location and number of unerupted teeth.

Natal Teeth

Premature eruption of teeth or teeth like structures that are present at birth. They are hyper mobile because of their limited root development. Teeth may be conical or may be normal in size and shape and opaque yellow-brownish in color (Fig. 1.38). Teeth appear to be attached to a small mass

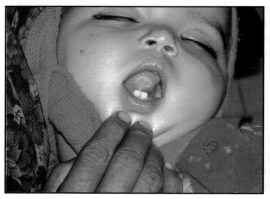

Fig. 1.38: Natal teeth seen in lower anterior region.
Also note the ulcer seen ventral surface of tongue

of soft tissue. Some teeth are so much mobile that there is danger of displacement and possible aspiration and in this case, removal is indicated.

STRUCTURE OF TEETH

Amelogenesis Imperfecta

It is also called as *'hereditary enamel dysplasia'*, *'hereditary brown enamel'* and *'hereditary brown opalescent teeth'*.

It can be *Hypoplastic type* (there is defective for-mation of enamel matrix) *Hypocalcification type* (there is defective mineralization of formed matrix) *hypomaturation type* (in this enamel crystal lattice remains immature).

Hypoplastic type (Fig. 1.39)—it appears as thin enamel on teeth that do not contact with each other mesiodistally. Horizontal rows of depressions or one large hypoplastic area with hypocalcification adjacent to and below the hypoplastic area is found.

Hypocalcified type—the enamel is so soft that it may be lost soon after eruption, leaving crown composed of only dentin. Enamel has cheesy consistency and can be scraped from dentin with an instrument or penetrated easily by dental explorer.

Hypomaturation type—the enamel can be pierced by an explorer point under firm pressure and can be lost by chipping away from the underlying, normal appearing dentin.

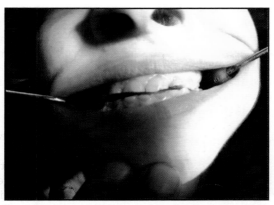

Fig. 1.39: Hypocalcified type of amelogenesis imperfecta showing only dentin due to loss of enamel

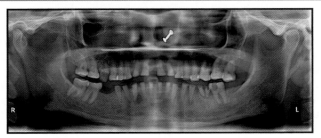

Fig. 1.40: Missing enamel resulting in squarish type of crown

Snow capped teeth—in this condition varying amount of enamel on incisal or occlusal aspect of crown is present and has opaque white appearances. Opacity may be solid or flecked and may involve enamel surface. Pattern of defect on teeth anterior to the posterior teeth resemble that which would be obtained when *'dipped into white paints'*.

Radiologically squarish type of crown being devoid of the normal mesial and distal contours (Fig. 1.40). The normal enamel cap is missing and in its place, there is thin and opaque layer of enamel.

Cosmetic improvement should be done.

Enamel Hypoplasia

It is an incomplete or defective formation of organic enamel matrix. Local and systemic factors that interfere with the normal matrix formation can cause enamel surface defects and irregularities. It can occur due to nutritional deficiency, exanthematous disease, congenital syphilis, hypocalcemia, birth injury, local infection, trauma, fluoride, tetracycline and chronic lead poisoning.

Drinking water that contains in excess of 1 PPM (part per million) fluoride can affect the ameloblasts during the tooth formation stage and can cause the clinical entity called as 'mottled enamel' (Fig. 1.41). It is due to disturbance in tooth formation caused by excessive intake of fluoride, during the formative period of dentition. It frequently becomes stained as unsightly yellow to brown color, (Fig. 1.42) which is caused by coloring agents from food, medicine and by disintegration of the increase protein contain in the hypomineralized parts of the enamel.

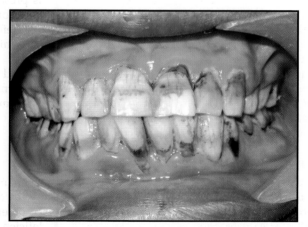

Fig. 1.41: Hypoplasia due to fluoride (*Courtesy*: Dr Abhishek Soni, Lecturer, Periodontia, VSPM Dental College and Research Center, Nagpur, India)

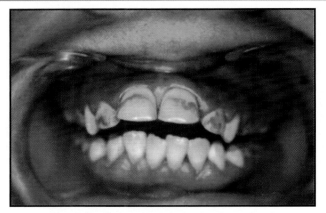

Fig. 1.42: Enamal hypoplasia showing yellow
to brown color discoloration

Radiologically extensive lesion appears as a series of rounded dark shadows crossing the tooth in straight lines (Fig. 1.43).

It is managed by bleaching with 30 percent H_2O_2 (hydrogen peroxide)—this technique is enhanced by micro-abrasion or grinding of the surface layer.

Dentinogenesis Imperfecta

There are various names for dentinogenesis imperfecta like *'hereditary opalescent dentin'* and *'odontogenesis imperfecta'*. It can be *Shield type I* (dentinogenesis imperfecta always occurs with osteogenesis imperfecta), *Shield type II* (it does not occur in association with osteogenesis imperfecta) and

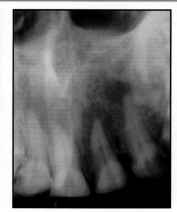

Fig. 1.43: Enamel hypoplasia showing absence of enamel on incisors with periapical pathology (*Courtesy*: Dr Amit Parate, Lecturer, Oral Medicine and Radiology, GDCH Nagpur, India)

shield type III (it has got shell teeth appearances and multiple pulp exposure).

Color of teeth may vary from brownish violet to yellowish brown (Fig. 1.44). Amber translucency of both primary and permanent dentition may be seen. Enamel may be lost and dentin undergoes rapid attrition. Usual scalloping of dentinoenamel junction is absent. The neck of teeth suddenly narrows down. The appearance of crowns may be described as *'dumpy'*.

Radiologically constriction of cervical portion of tooth that imparts bullous appearance (Fig. 1.45). Partial or complete obliteration of pulp chamber. Pulp obliteration may

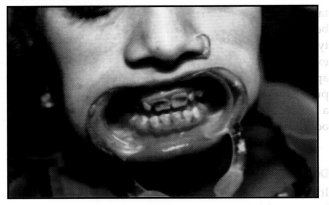

Fig. 1.44: Exposed dentin, stained dark brown suggestive of dentinogenesis imperfecta

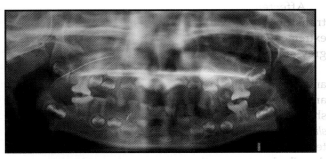

Fig. 1.45: Radiograph showing bulbous crown with constriction in the cervical region

take place before or after eruption of teeth. Root canals may be absent or thread like or may be blunted. In Brandywine type, enamel of tooth appears normal, while the dentin is extremely thin and the pulp chambers are enormous. Teeth appear as *'shell teeth'*. In some cases the radicular portion of pulp cavities is very narrow, while the pulp chambers have a bulbous expansion terminating in a point deep to the occlusal aspect which resembles *'flame'*.

Cast metal crown should be given.

Dentin Dysplasia

It is a rare disturbance of dentin formation, characterized by normal but atypical dentin formation, with abnormal pulp morphology. It can be radicular or coronal types. It is transmitted as autosomal dominant trait.

Affected teeth are occasionally slightly amber and translucent. Malalignment and malpositioning due to extreme mobility. Primary teeth with yellow, brown, bluish, grey-amber translucent appearances.

Radiologically tooth has short roots with sharp conical and apical constriction (Fig. 1.46). Pulp chamber and canals are obliterated before eruption and appears as half moon shaped. Obliteration of pulp chamber produce *'crescent shaped'* pulp remnants (Fig. 1.46). In coronal type permanent teeth exhibit large chamber in coronal portion which is described as *'thistle tube'* in shape which is due to radiating extension of pulp chamber.

It is managed by prosthetic replacement.

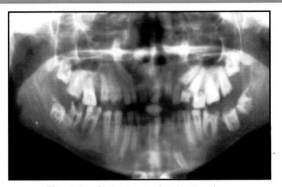

Fig. 1.46: Obliteration of pulp chambers
indicating dentin dysplasia

GROWTH OF TEETH

Embedded and Impacted Teeth

Embedded teeth are those which are unerupted, usually because of lack of eruptive force. *Impacted teeth* are those prevented from erupting by some physical barrier in eruption path (Fig. 1.47).

It is caused by lack of space, rotation of tooth bud, and systemic disease like Osteopetrosis, ectodermal dysplasia, cleidocranial dysostosis, rickets and cretinism can be associated with impactions.

Teeth may be impacted distally, mesially, horizontally, etc (Figs 1.48 and 1.49). Periodontal pocket formation and subsequent infections may occur. Because of location, impacted tooth may cause resorption of roots of adjacent teeth.

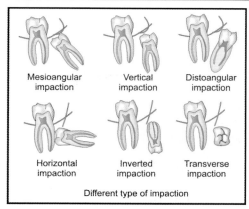

Fig. 1.47: Different types of impaction seen in oral cavity

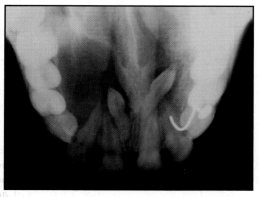

Fig. 1.48: Inverted impacted canine seen in upper anterior region

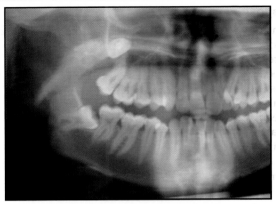

Fig. 1.49: Vertical impacted tooth in the sinus and mesioangular impacted third molar

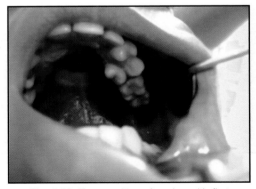

Fig. 1.50: Transposition of canine with first premolar left upper posterior region

Transposition

Tooth may be found occupying an unusual position in relation to other teeth, in the dental arch, i.e. two teeth apparently exchanging their position (Fig. 1.50).

Teeth often exchange their positions. Permanent canine is most often involved, with its position interchanged with lateral incisor. Second premolar is infrequently found between first and second molar. Transposition of central and lateral incisor is rare. Transposition does not occur in primary dentition.

It can be recognized on radiograph by the unusual sequence of teeth in dental arch (Fig. 1.51).

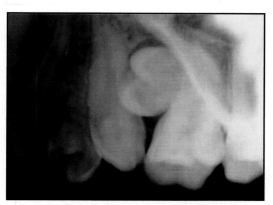

Fig. 1.51: Transposition of canine with premolar

Keratotic and Nonkeratotic Lesion

NORMAL VARIATION

Leukoedema

It is an abnormality of the buccal mucosa, which clinically resembles early leukoplakia. It is cause by use of tobacco, racial and related to poor oral hygiene.

Buccal mucosa retains the normal softness and flexibility but exhibits grayish white, slightly folded opalescent appearance (Fig. 2.1) that is described as epithelium covered with diffuse edematous film or *velvetlike veil*. It can be eliminated by the stretching and scraping of mucosa but reestablishes itself almost immediately.

No treatment is necessary.

Fordyce Granule

A Fordyce granule is a developmental anomaly characterized by heterotrophic collection of sebaceous glands at various sites in oral cavity which is covered with intact mucosa.

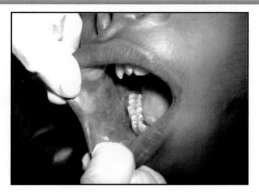

Fig. 2.1: Folded opalescent appearance seen in case of leukoedema

They appear as small yellow spots, projecting slightly above the surface of tissue. Sometime they may occur in clusters and may form plaque like lesions. It increases rapidly in number at puberty and continues to increase throughout adult life.

If it causes disfigurement then surgical removal can be done.

Linea Alba

Linea Alba refers to the line of keratinization, found on the buccal mucosa parallel to the line of occlusion expanding to a triangular area inside each labial comissure. (Fig. 2.2)

It is caused by variation in dietary and oral hygiene practice, frequent frictional contact with food and teeth.

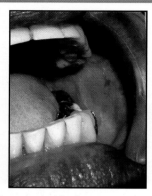

Fig. 2.2: Increased white line seen at occlusal plane which is giving triangular shape at retromolar area

NONKERATOTIC WHITE LESIONS

Habitual Cheek or Lip Biting

It is also called as *'Morsicato buccarum.'* It is produced by frequent and repeated rubbing, sucking or chewing movements that abrade the surface of a wide area of lip or cheek mucosa without producing discrete ulceration (Fig. 2.3).

Usually there is opaque white appearance and is homogenous. In some cases, there is macerated and reddened area usually with patch of partly detached surface epithelium (Fig. 2.4). In some cases, contused margins present with transient whitish tags of necrotic tissue around the ulcer.

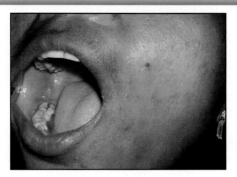

Fig. 2.3: Chronic cheek biting occur in retromolar area due to trauma from third molar

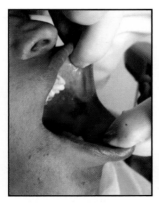

Fig. 2.4: Habitual cheek biting presented as macerated and reddened area on the cheek mucosa

Thermal Burns

It can be caused by hot food, beverages is present, pain which last for short duration. It may produce coagulation necrosis of superficial tissue that appears whitish. In some cases, there may be frank ulceration and stripping of mucosa. Red area is tender on palpation. Surface layer of epithelium is desquamated.

Pizza Burns

It is whitish grey or ulcerated lesions of the middle third of the hard palate. These also present superficial necrosis and ulceration due to combination of heat of the cheese and its adhesion to epithelium (Fig. 2.5).

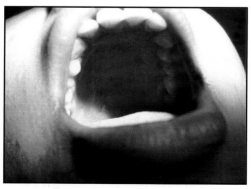

Fig. 2.5: Pizza burn showing ulceration at junction of soft and hard palate and with whitish desquamation

Radiation Mucositis

It is secondary to therapeutic radiation of head and neck cancer. It develops towards the end of the 1st week of therapy. It occurs if radiation given in excess of 3500 to 4000 rads. There is redness of oral mucosa followed by pseudomembrane formation with large area of oral mucosa covered with grayish, white slough alternating with areas of severe ulceration (Fig. 2.6).

It is managed by a soothing mouth rinse.

Candidiasis

It is also called as *'candidosis'*. Candidiasis is the disease caused by infection with yeast like fungus *Candida albicans*.

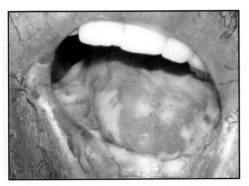

Fig. 2.6: Generalized mucositis involving tongue and angular cheilitis occur in patient who receive radiotherapy

CLASSIFICATION

Oral Candidiasis

Acute

- Acute pseudomembranous candidiasis (thrush)
- Acute atrophic candidiasis (antibiotics sore mouth)

Chronic

- Chronic atrophic candidiasis
  - Denture stomatitis
  - Median rhomboidal glossitis
  - Angular cheilitis
- ID reaction
- Chronic hyperplastic candidiasis.

Chronic Mucocutaneous Candidiasis

- Familial CMC
- Localized CMC
- Diffuse CMC
- Candidiasis endocrinopathy syndrome.

Extraoral Candidiasis

- Oral candidiasis associated with extraoral lesions orofacial and intertriginous sites (candidal vulvovaginitis, intertriginous candidiasis)
- Gastrointestinal candidiasis
- Candida hypersensitivity syndrome.

Systemic Candidiasis

- Mainly affect the eye, kidney and skin.

Thrush

It is the superficial infection of upper layer of oral mucous membrane and results in formation of patchy white plaque or flecks on mucosal surface.

In neonates, oral lesions start between the 6th and 10th day after birth. Infection is contracted from the maternal vaginal canal, where *Candida albicans* flourishes during the pregnancy. The lesions in infants are described as soft white or bluish white, adherent patches on oral mucosa which may extent to circumoral tissue (Fig. 2.7). They are painless. They may be removed with little difficulty.

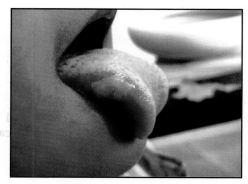

Fig. 2.7: Soft white lesion seen in candidiasis in children (*Courtesy:* Revent Chole, Lecturer, People Dental College, Bhopal, India)

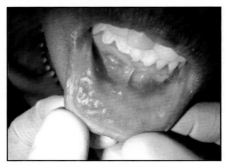

Fig. 2.8: Candidiasis occurring on lip as white plaque which can be removed easily (*Courtesy:* Revent Chole, Lecturer, People Dental College, Bhopal, India)

In adults prodormal symptom like rapid onset of bad taste is present. Patient may complain of burning sensation with history of dryness of the mouth. Inflammation, erythema, and painful eroded areas may be associated with this disease. Sometimes typical, pearly white or bluish white plaque is present. Mucosa adjacent to it appears red and moderately swollen. Lesions are relatively inconspicuous (Fig. 2.8). White patches are easily wiped out with wet gauze, which leaves either a normal or erythematous area or atrophic area.

Acute Atrophic Candidiasis

It is also called as 'antibiotics sore mouth'. When the white plaque of pseudomembranous candidiasis is removed, often red atrophic and painful mucosa remains.

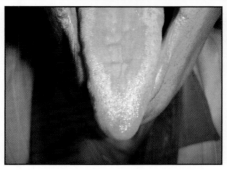

Fig. 2.9: Acute atrophic candidiasis showing red erythematous area (*Courtesy:* Revent Chole, Lecturer, People Dental College, Bhopal, India)

In this type, lesions appear as red or erythematous rather than white, thus resembling the pseudo-membranous type in which white membrane has been wiped off (Fig. 2.9). Patient usually described vague pain or a burning sensation. Careful examination reveals a few white thickened foci that rub off leaving a painful surface.

Chronic Hyperplastic Candidiasis

It is also called as *'candidal leukoplakia'* because of its firm presentation as firm and adherent white patches occurring in the oral mucosa. The majority of these patients are heavy smokers.

Candidal leukoplakia is extremely chronic form of oral candidiasis in which firm, and white leathery plaques are found (Fig. 2.10). Lesions may persist without any symptoms

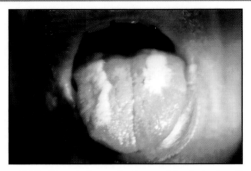

Fig. 2.10: Chronic hyperplastic candidiasis having firm leathery appearance

for years. It does not rub off with lateral pressure. Lesion range from slightly white to dense white with cracks and fissures occasionally present (Fig. 2.11). The borders are often vague, which mimic the appearance of epithelial dysplasia.

ID Reaction

A person with chronic *Candida* infection may develop secondary response characterized by localized or generalized sterile vesicopapular rash that is believed to be allergic response to *Candida* antigen (also called as monolids).

Chronic Atrophic Candidiasis

It is also called as *'chronic atrophic candidiasis'*. It is common clinical manifestation of erythematous candidiasis. It occurs

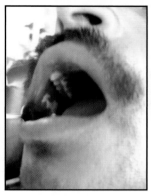

Fig. 2.11: Candidial leukoplakia on right buccal mucosa (*Courtesy:* Revent Chole, Lecturer, People Dental College, Bhopal, India)

due to tissue invasion but organism effect of fungal toxin hypersensitivity to fungus.

It is usually found under complete denture and partial denture. It exhibits patchy distribution. There is soreness and dryness of mouth.

Palatal tissue is bright red edematous and granular. The redness of mucosa is rather sharply outlined and restricted to the tissue actually in contact with the denture (Fig. 2.12). The multiple pinpoint foci of hyperemia usually involving the maxilla frequently occur.

Topical Treatment

Clotrimazole (one oral troche, 10 mg tablet) 1% gentian violet, nystatin preparations (nystatin vaginal tablets nystatin oral

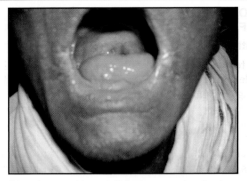

Fig. 2.12: Chronic atrophic candidiasis occurring in denture wearer (*Courtesy:* Revent Chole, Lecturer, People Dental College, Bhopal, India)

pastille (available as a 200,000-unit oral pastille, one or two pastilles dissolved slowly in the mouth five times a day).

Rinses

Mycostatin rinses for 7 to 10 days 3 to 4 times a day. 0.2% chlorhexidine solution, use of 1% chlorhexidine gel in denture stomatitis.

Systemic Treatment

Nystatin (250 mg tds for 2 week followed by 1 troche per day for third week), ketoconazole (200 mg tablet) fluconazole (100 mg tablet taken once daily for 2 weeks), itraconazole (100 mg capsules).

KERATOTIC WHITE LESIONS WITH NO DEFINITE PRECANCEROUS POTENTIAL

Traumatic Keratosis

It refer to isolated area of thickened whitish oral mucosa that is clearly related to identifiable local irritant and resolves following elimination of irritant.

It is cause by *local irritants* like ill fitting denture, sharp clasp and rough edges of restoration and heavy cigarettes smoking (Fig. 2.13).

Glassblower's white patch—It is variant of traumatic keratosis affecting the cheek and lips, which occur in glass factory.

Upon removal of the offending agent, the lesion should resolve within 2 weeks. Biopsies should be performed on lesions that do not heal to rule out a dysplastic lesion.

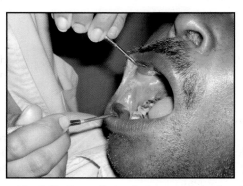

Fig. 2.13: Traumatic keratosis seen at cheek mucosa due to sharp cusp

Psoriasis

It is common a dermatological disease characterized by white, scaly papules and plaque on an erythematous base that preferentially affects the extremities and scalp.

It is transmitted as simple dominant trait. It is caused by infection (β-hemolytic streptococcal infection), metabolic disturbances, endocrine dysfunction, drugs (antimalarials, β-blocker and lithium). Mental anxiety, stress and trauma can increase severity of the disease.

It is characterized by occurrence of small sharply defined, dry papules each covered by delicate silvery scale which appear as resembling a thin layer of mica (Fig. 2.14). *Auspitz's sign* (if the deep scale is removed one or more

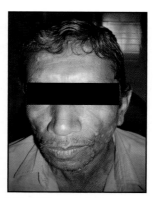

Fig. 2.14: White scaly lesion seen on the face of patient having psoriasis

bleeding points are seen) is seen. Papules are enlarged at periphery and may form large plaques which are roughly symmetrical. After removal of scale the surface of skin is red and dusky in appearance.

Oral lesions are reported on lip, buccal mucosa, palate, gingiva and floor of mouth. They appear as plaques, silvery, scaly lesions with an erythematous base.

It is managed by *emollients, dithranol* (gold standard therapy), tar, calcipotriol (vitamin D agonist), *retinoid, corticosteroids, ultraviolet light, PUVA therapy* (psoralens) and *systemic treatment* (methotrexate, oral retinoid and cyclosporin).

Oral Premalignant Lesions and Conditions

Oral pre-cancer is distinguished into:

PRE-CANCEROUS LESION

It is defined as a morphologically altered tissue in which cancer is more likely to occur, than its apparently normal counter parts. For example:
- Leukoplakia
- Erythroplakia
- Mucosal changes associated with smoking habits
- Carcinoma *in situ*
- Bowen disease
- Actinic keratosis, cheilitis and elastosis.

PRE-CANCEROUS CONDITION

It is defined as a generalized state or condition associated with significantly increased risk for cancer development. For example:
- Oral submucus fibrosis (OSMF)
- Syphilis
- Sideropenic dysplasia

- Oral lichen planus
- Dyskeratosis congenita
- Lupus erythematosus.

Leukoplakia

The term leukoplakia originates from two Greek words-leuko, i.e. white and plakia i.e. patch. It is defined as any white patch on mucosa, which cannot be rubbed or scraped off and which cannot be attributed to any other diagnosable disease.

By Who

It is a whitish patch or plaque that cannot be characterized, clinically or pathologically, as any other disease and which is not associated with any other physical or chemical causative agent except the use of tobacco.

It can be homogeneous (completely whitish lesion), non-homogeneous (can be nodular, verrucous, ulcerated and erythroleukoplakia). It can be leukoplakia simplex (a uniform raised plaque formation, varying in size, with regular edges. It corresponds to homogeneous type of leukoplakia), Leukoplakia erosive (a lesion with slightly raised, rounded, red and/or whitish excrescence, that may be described as granules or nodules) and Leukoplakia verrucosa (verrucous proliferation raised above the mucosal surface).

It is caused by tobacco which can be smokeless tobacco (chewable tobacco and oral use of snuff) and smoking tobacco (cigar, cigarette, bidi and pipe).

Sharp staging of leukoplakia
- Stage I—Earliest lesion-non-palpable, faintly translucent, white discoloration.
- Stage II—Localized or diffuse, slightly elevated plaque of irregular outline. It is opaque white and may have fine granular texture.
- Stage III—Thickened white lesion showing induration and fissuring.

Homogeneous

It is also called as leukoplakia simplex. It accounts for 84% of cases. Usually, localized lesions of extensive white patches present a relatively consistent pattern throughout (Fig. 3.1). It is characterized by raised plaque formation consisting of single or group of plaques varying in size with

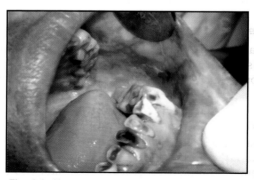

Fig. 3.1: Homogeneous leukoplakia showing white patch on left buccal mucosa

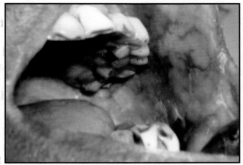

Fig. 3.2: Leukoplakia on left buccal mucosa extending from angle of mouth. It also show discoloration on buccal mucosa due to tobacco habit

irregular edges (Fig. 3.2). They are usually white in color but may be yellowish white or yellow.

Ulcerated Leukoplakia

It is characterized by red area, which at times exhibit yellowish areas of fibrin, giving the appearance of ulceration. White patches are present at the periphery of the lesion.

Nodular Leukoplakia

It is also called as 'leukoplakia erosiva' or 'speckled leukoplakia'. A mixed red white lesion is seen in which small keratotic nodules are scattered over an atrophic patch of oral mucosa. Nodules may be pinhead sized or even larger. It has got a high malignant potential.

Verrucous Leukoplakia

It is also called as 'leukoplakia verrucosa'. It is characterized by verrucous proliferation above the mucosal surface. It is a white lesion with a broken up surface due to multiple papillary projections that may be heavily keratinized (Fig. 3.3). It is slow growing, persistent and irreversible. In the course of time erythematous component may develop in the lesion. Later, it becomes exophytic and wart like and transforms into a lesion that is clinically and microscopically identical to verrucous carcinoma or squamous cell carcinoma.

Extensive lesions of verrucous leukoplakia are called 'oral florid papillomatosis'.

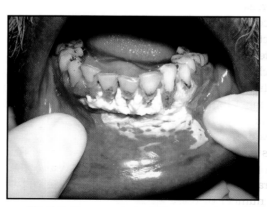

Fig. 3.3: Verrucous leukoplakia seen in lower anterior region as exophytic growth

It is managed by elimination of etiological factor, vitamin therapy (Vitamin A + vitamin E, 13-cis-retinoic acid), antioxidant therapy (B-carotene), vitamin A palmitate, nystatin therapy, vitamin B complex, anti-mycotic preparation.

Surgically it is managed by conventional surgery, cryosurgery, fulguration (electrocautery and electrosurgery), LASER (light amplification of stimulated emission of radiation).

Erythroplakia

It is also called as erythroplasia of Queyrat. Erythroplakia is a persistent velvety red patch. Reddish color results from absence of surface keratin layer and due to presence of connective tissue papillae containing enlarged capillaries projected close to the surface.

A chronic red mucosal macule which cannot be given any other specific diagnostic name and cannot be attributed to traumatic, vascular or inflammatory causes.

It can be homogeneous, erythroplakia interspersed with patches of leukoplakia, and speckled or granular.

It is asymptomatic. It is nonelevated, red macule or patch on an epithelial surface. The exact cause of the red appearance is unknown, but may be related to an increase in the number of underlying blood vessels through which the blood flows, which in turn may be secondary to localized inflammatory or immunological responses caused by the dysplastic, i.e. 'foreign,' epithelial cells. In some cases, the color may result from a lack of surface keratin or extreme thinness of the epithelium.

Homogeneous Form

It commonly found on buccal mucosa and soft palate and rarely on tongue and floor of mouth. Homogeneous form appears as a bright red, soft, velvety lesion with straight or scalloped, well-demarcated margins (Fig. 3.4). It is often quite extensive in size.

It usually quite sharply demarcated from the surrounding pink mucosa and its surface is typically smooth and regular in coloration.

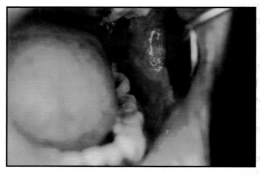

Fig. 3.4: Erythroplakia presenting as bright red patch on buccal mucosa. It has got well defined margin

Granular or Speckled Form

These are soft, red lesions that are slightly elevated with irregular outlines and granular or finely nodular surface speckled with tiny white plaques.

Erythroleukoplakia

It is quite common to see erythroplakia admixed with or adjacent to leukoplakia in mouth. Erythroplakia interspersed with patches of leukoplakia in which erythematous areas are irregular and often not as bright as homogeneous form, are most frequently seen on tongue and floor of mouth. The borders may be well circumscribed or blend impercibly with surrounding oral mucosa.

Since erythroplakia is so closely correlated with severe dysplasia, carcinoma *in situ* and invasive carcinoma, incisional biopsy is especially indicated. Destructive techniques such as laser ablation, electrocoagulation and cryotherapy have also proved to be effective.

Carcinoma *in Situ*

It is also called as 'intraepithelial carcinoma'. Severe dysplastic changes in a white lesion indicate considerable risk of development of cancer. The more severe grade of dysplasia merges with the condition known as carcinoma *in situ*. It is more common on skin but can also occur on mucous membrane.

Appearance of the lesion may be like leukoplakia, like erythroplakia. It may be a combination of leukoplakia and erythroplakia, ulcerated lesion, ulcerated and white lesion, red and ulcerated lesion or may be non-specific.

Lesion may be surgical excise, cauterized and even exposed to solid carbon dioxide.

Bowen's Disease

It is localized 'intra-epidermoid carcinoma' that may progress to invasive carcinoma over many years, which is characterized by progressive scaly or crusted plaque like lesion.

It is cause by sun exposure and arsenic ingestion.

It appears as slowing enlarging erythematous patches. There is a red and slightly scaly area on the skin, which eventually enlarges and turns into white or yellowish lesion. When these scales are removed it produced a granular surface without bleeding.

Use of freezing technique, diathermy, cauterization, radiotherapy or application of cytotoxic drugs.

ORAL LESION ASSOCIATED WITH USE OF TOBACCO

Smoker's Palate or Stomatitis Nicotina

It is seen in persons who are heavy pipe and cigar smokers and it is most common in males. It is most commonly seen in reverse smoking habit.

The palate develops diffuse, grayish-white, thickened, multinodular papular appearance. There is small red spot in the center of each tiny nodule, representing a dilated and sometimes partially occluded orifice of an accessory palatal salivary gland duct around which inflammatory cell infiltration is prominent (Fig. 3.5). The epithelium around the duct shows excessive thickening and keratinization. Fissures and crack may appear, producing a wrinkled, irregular surface (Fig. 3.6).

It can be mild (red, dot like opening on blanched area), (Fig. 3.7) moderate (well define elevation with central umbilication) and severe (marked by papules of 5 mm or more with umbilication of 2-3 mm).

Cigarette Smoker's Lip Lesion

They are generally flat or slightly elevated nodular white lesion on one or both lips, corresponding to the site at which

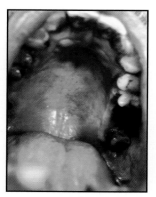

Fig. 3.5: Smoke palate with reddened mucosa (*Courtesy:* Revent Chole, Lecturer, People Dental College, Bhopal, India)

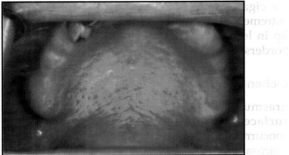

Fig. 3.6: Stomatitis nicotina showing red dot like opening on blanched area

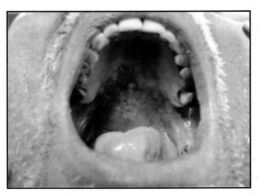

Fig. 3.7: Opening of salivary gland seen red center surrounded focal thickening

the cigarette is held and apparently smoked down to an extremely short length. Increased redness and stippling of lip in localized area. It has elliptical, circular or irregular borders.

Lichen Planus

Erasmus Wilson described it in 1869. Various mucosal surfaces may be involved, either independently or concurrently, with cutaneous involvement or serially. Oral mucosa is frequently involved. It is a probable pre-cancerous condition. Lichen planus is a common inflammatory disease of the skin presenting with characteristic violaceous, polygonal, pruritic papules. The disease may also affect the mucosa, hair and nails.

It is relatively common dermatological disorder occurring on skin (Fig. 3.8) and oral mucous membrane and refers to lace-like pattern produced by symbolic algae and fungal colonies on the surface of rocks in nature (lichens). It is caused by cell mediated immune response (haptens, certain drug or dental material), conventional antigen or super-antigen of oral microbial origin can induce cell mediated immune response resulting in sub-epithelial T cell infiltration of the site in oral mucosa with cytokine generation HSP-60 and C 1/10 expression by basal keratinocytes), auto-immunity, immunodeficiency, genetic factors, infec-tion, drugs. A relationship of lichen planus with stress is quoted and neurogenic basis is suggested.

Oral lichen planus has shown association with tobacco habit. Chewers of tobacco and betel have increased prevalence of oral lichen planus.

It can be reticular, papular, plaque, atrophic, erythematous, ulcerative, hypertrophic, erosive, bullous, hypertrophied, annular, actinic, follicular and linear type.

Syndrome associated with lichen planus are Grinspan syndrome (Lichen planus, diabetes mellitus, vascular hypertension) and Graham little syndrome

The chief complains is usually of intense pruritus. The itching associated with LP usually provokes rubbing of the lesions, rather than scratching. The lesions have a characteristic violet hue (Fig. 3.8). They are flat-topped, shiny, polygonal papules and plaques. The surface is dry with thin, adherent scales.

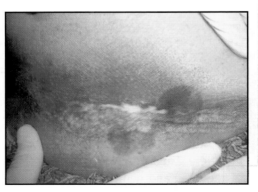

Fig. 3.8: Skin lesion seen in lichen planus

Six P of lichen planus - six 'p's characterize the lesions LP: they are planar, polygonal, purple, pruritic, papules and plaques.

Wickham's Striae

These are very fine grayish lines which cover the papules (Fig. 3.9). Koebner phenomenon—fresh lesions may appear on scratch marks or at sites of other non-specific trauma.

Orally patient may report with burning sensation of oral mucosa. Oral lesion is characterized by radiating white and gray velvety thread like papules in a linear, angular or retiform arrangement forming typical lacy, reticular patterns, rings and streaks over the buccal mucosa and to a lesser extent on the lip, tongue and palate.

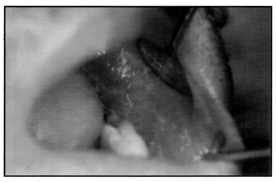

Fig. 3.9: Reticular type of lichen planus showing fine whitish line

Reticular Type

Most common form and it is mostly bilateral. Consists of slightly elevated fine whitish lines that produce lace like pattern of fine radiating lines, called as Wickham's striae (Fig. 3.10). The lesion may present radiating white thread like papules in a linear, annular or retiform arrangement. A tiny white dot is frequently present at the intersection of white lines (Fig. 3.11).

Papular

Whitish elevated lesions of 0.5 to 1 mm in size, well seen on keratinized areas of oral mucosa. Papules are spaced apart, still close enough to give pebbled white or gray color. Most often, papules are seen at the periphery of reticular pattern.

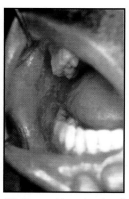

Fig. 3.10: Wickham striae showing fine grayish line in retromolar area in lichen planus

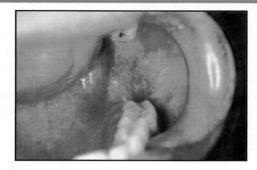

Fig. 3.11: Reticular type of lichen planus seen in retromolar area

Plaque

Seen on dorsum of tongue and buccal mucosa. It consists of either pearly white or grayish white plaque. Such plaques generally range from slightly elevated and smooth to slightly irregular form.

Atrophic Form

Appears as smooth, red, poorly defined area, often but not always, with peripheral striae evident. At the margins of atrophic zones, whitish keratotic striae are usually evident, radiating peripherally and blending into surrounding mucosa. The gingiva tends to show patchy distribution over all the four quadrants in a relatively symmetrical pattern. It is always symptomatic with complain of pain and burning in the areas of involvement.

Bullous Form

It consists of vesicles and bullae which are short lived. These upon rupturing, leave an ulcerated extremely uncomfortable surface. The most common site is buccal mucosa especially into posterior and lateral margins of tongue. It is often associated with striated or keratotic component.

Hypertrophic Form

It appears as well circumscribed, elevated white lesion resembling leukoplakia (Fig. 3.12).

Annular Form

Appears as round or ovoid, white outline with either pink or reddish pink center (Fig. 3.13).

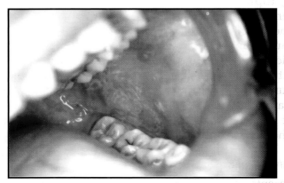

Fig. 3.12: Hypertrophic variety showing elevated lesion

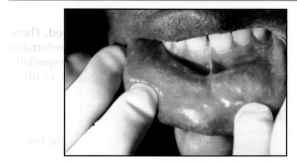

Fig. 3.13: Annular type of lichen planus seen on labial mucosa

It is managed by steroids. Small and moderately sized painful lesions can be treated with beclomethasone dipropionate spray, triamcinolone acetonide in gel or cream base, topical and intralesional routes are used when systemic steroids are contraindicated. Injection triamcinolone acetonide 10 mg/ml was also used in patients with serious complain, in a dose of 0.1 ml/cm². Topical application of fluocinolone acetonide for 4 weeks is also effective in curing the disease. Topical application of antifungal agent, vitamin A (Retinoid) analogue, Retinoids, topical vitamin A acid cream (0.1%).

It can be treated by cyclosporin, surgical therapy, psychotherapy, dapsone therapy, PUVA therapy.

Erosive Lichen Planus

It presents as chronic multiple oral mucosal ulcers, which occur when there is extensive degeneration of basal cell layer of epithelium.

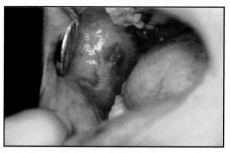

Fig. 3.14: Erosive lichen planus showing ulcerated lesions with lacy pattern at periphery

It is caused by drug therapy like NSAIDs, hydrochlorothiazide, penicillamine, angiotensin converting enzyme inhibitors, chronic hepatitis, dental restoration, graft versus host disease and emotional stress can lead to erosive lichen planus.

There is complain of burning sensation and pain. After rupture of vesicles, eroded or frankly ulcerated lesion are seen which appears as a raw painful areas (Fig. 3.14). Lacy white pattern may be present. Eroded and frankly ulcerated lesions are irregular in size and shape and appear as raw and painful areas. The surface is generally granular and brightly erythematous and may bleed upon slight provocation or manipulation.

Oral Submucus Fibrosis

It is a chronic and high-risk precancerous condition. Schwartz (1952) was the first person to bring this condition again into limelight. He described the condition as *'atrophica idiopathic mucosae oris'*. It also called as idiopathic scleroderma of mouth, idiopathic palatal fibrosis and sclerosing stomatitis.

It is an insidious, chronic disease affecting any part of the oral cavity and sometimes pharynx. Although occasionally preceded by and/or associated with vesicle formation, it is always associated with juxtaepithelial inflammatory reaction followed by fibroelastic changes of lamina propria, with epithelial atrophy leading to stiffness of oral mucosa and causing trismus and inability to eat.

The disease is very common in India, Indian subcontinent and other Asian people It is caused by *chillies* (capsicum annum and capsicum frutescence), *Tobacco, lime, Betel nut* (areca nut). It is also caused by nutritional deficiency, defective iron metabolism, bacterial infections (streptococcal toxicity, Klebsiella rhinoscleromatis), collagen disease (scleroderma, rheumatoid arthritis, Duputreyen's contracture and intestinal fibrosis), immunological disorders, genetic susceptibility and altered salivary composition.

The onset of the condition is insidious and is often of 2 to 5 yrs of duration. The most common initial symptom is burning sensation of oral mucosa, aggravated by spicy food, followed by either hyper salivation or dryness of mouth. Vesiculation, ulceration, pigmentation, recurrent stomatitis and defective gustatory sensation have also been indicated as early symptoms.

Gradual stiffening of the oral mucosa occurs in few years after the initial symptoms appear (Fig. 3.15). This leads to

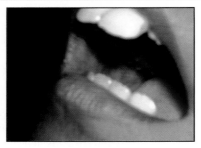

Fig. 3.15: Oral submucus fibrosis seen in young patient.
Note the pale mucosa

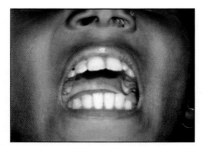

Fig. 3.16: Oral submucus fibrosis involving soft palate

inability to open the mouth. Later on patients experience difficulty in protruding the tongue. When the fibrosis extends to pharynx (Fig. 3.16) and esophagus, the patient may experience difficulty in swallowing the food.

The most common and earliest sign is blanching of mucosa, caused by impairment of local vascularity. The blanched mucosa becomes slightly opaque and white. The whitening often takes place in spots so that the mucosa acquires a marble like appearance. Blanching may be localized or diffuse, involving greater part of the oral mucosa or reticular, in which blanching consists of blanched area with intervening clinically normal mucosa, giving it a lace like appearance. As disease progresses the mucosa becomes stiff and vertical fibrous bands appear there. It can show ulceration showing sign of malignant transformation (Fig. 3.17)

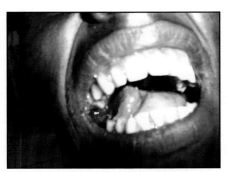

Fig. 3.17: Oral submucus fibrosis showing ulceration indicate malignancy transformation

The preventive measure should be in the form of stoppage of habit, which can be encouraged through public education. Affected patients should be explained about the disease and its possible malignant potential. Improvement in clinical features like gradual increase in inter-incisal opening has been observed in most of the patients who discontinue the habit.

Medicinal treatment consists of iodine-B-complex preparation, m*ethyltrioxyethyl iodomine, Vitamins and steroids, placental extract.*

Lupus Erythematosus

It is characterized by presence of abnormal antibodies and immune complex. It can be d*iscoid lupus erythematosus* (confined to skin and mucosa) and s*ystemic lupus erythematosus* (if multiorgan involvement occurs).

It is caused by g*enetic predisposition, immunological abnormality possibly mediated by viral infection, autoimmune disease, deposition of antigen–antibody complexes, endocrine* (high incidence in females in pregnancy), and *biochemical increase* in excretion of metabolic products, particularly tyrosine and phenylalanine, in certain SLE patient.

Discoid Type

It is a circumscribed, slightly elevated, white patch that may be surrounded by red telangiectatic halo. Cutaneous lesions are slightly elevated, red or purple macules; that are often covered by gray or yellow adherent scales. Forceful removal of scale results in 'carpet track extension', which has dipped into enlarged pilosebaceous canals. Butterfly distribution on macular region and across the bridge of the nose. Orally it begins as erythematous area, sometimes slightly elevated, but more often depressed, usually with induration and typically with white spots. There may be burning and tenderness which may be intermittent or disappear if the lesion becomes inactive. The margins of the lesion are not sharply demarcated. Fine white striae radiate out from the margins.

Systemic Type

It is manifested by symptoms of fever and pain in the muscle and joints. It may present as itching or burning sensation as well as area of hyper-pigmentation. Severely intensifies after exposure to sunlight. The cutaneous lesion consists of erythematous patches on the face, which coalesce to form roughly symmetrical pattern over the cheeks and across the bridge of the nose, in a so called butterfly distribution. Skin lesions are widespread, bilateral with signs of acute inflammation.

This finding helps to differentiate between skin lesions of DLE and SLE. Involvement of various organs including kidneys and heart. Orally there is complain of burning sensation, xerostomia or soreness of mouth. Lesions similar to DLE, except that hyperemia, edema and extension of lesion is more pronounced. Greater tendency to bleed and petechiae, suspected ulcerations surrounded by red halo (Fig. 3.18). The lip lesions appear with central atrophic area

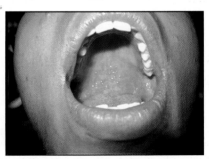

Fig. 3.18: Ulceration seen in soft palate area in systemic lupus erythematous

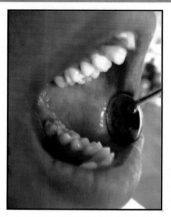

Fig. 3.19: Same patient having ulceration in buccal mucosa

with small white dots surrounded by keratinized border, which is composed of small radiating white striae. There is occasional ulceration of central area. The intraoral lesion is composed of a central depressed red atrophic area surrounded by 2 to 4 mm elevated (Fig. 3.19) keratotic zone that dissolves into small white lines.

It is treated by systemic corticosteroids therapy and should be managed by physician. Anti-malarial drugs can be used in some cases.

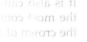

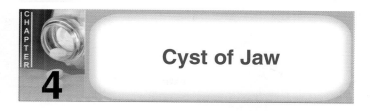

Cyst of Jaw

DENTIGEROUS CYST

It is also called as 'follicular cyst' or 'pericoronal cyst'. It is the most common type of odontogenic cyst which encloses the crown of the unerupted tooth by expansion of its follicle and is attached to the neck.

It is formed due to fluid accumulation in the layer of reduced enamel epithelium or between it and the crown of unerupted teeth.

Most commonly associated with mandibular third molars and maxillary canines which are most commonly impacted. They vary in size from a little more than the diameter of the involved crown to an expansion that causes progressive but painless enlargement of jaws and facial asymmetry (Fig. 4.1). Teeth adjacent to the developing cyst and involved teeth may get severely displaced and resorbed. There may be displacement of third molars to such an extent that it sometimes comes to lie compressed against the inferior border of the mandible.

Generally, it is painless but may be painful if it gets infected. When dentigerous cyst expands rapidly to

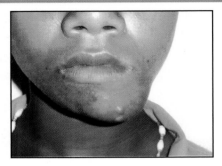

Fig. 4.1: Dentigerous cyst showing expansion of the jaw (*Courtesy: Dr Bhaskar Patle, Lecturer Oral Medicine and Radiology, SPDC, Wardha, India*)

compress sensory nerve it produces pain which may be referred to other sites and described as headache. In some cases pathological fracture can occur.

Cystic involvement of an unerupted third molar may result in hollowing out of the entire ramus extending up to the coronoid process and condyle as well as the body causing expansion of cortical plates.

Radiologically there is well-defined radiolucency usually associated with hyperostotic borders unless they are secondarily infected and is seen around an unerupted tooth (Fig. 4.2). Usually, it is unilocular but sometimes it may appear multilocular, this image is caused by ridges in the bony wall and not by the presence of bony septa. The bony margins are well-defined and sharp (Fig. 4.3). It may envelope the crown symmetrically, but it may expand

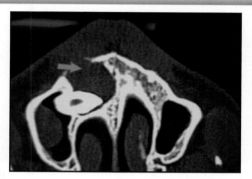

Fig. 4.2: CT scan of dentigerous cyst showing well-defined lesion (red arrow) with destruction of cortical plate

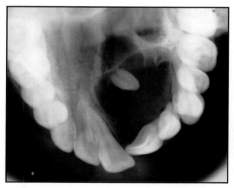

Fig. 4.3: Dentigerous cyst presented as envelopmental variety in relation with canine

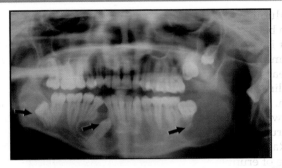

Fig. 4.4: Multiple dentigerous cyst (red arrow) seen in mandible

laterally from the crown. Associated tooth may be displaced in any direction (Fig. 4.4). It is usual for those unerupted teeth which become surrounded by the growing cyst to retain their follicle for a time at least, which serves to indicate that the tooth is actually outside the cyst.

Radiologically, it may be central variety (crown is enveloped symmetrically), lateral type (dilation of the follicle on one aspect of the crown), circumferential type (entire tooth appears to be enveloped by the cyst).

It is managed by surgical removal, marsupialization, and decompression. Complication includes ameloblastoma, mucoepidermoid carcinoma.

ERUPTION CYST

A specific type of cyst, which must be classified as a form of dentigerous cyst, is frequently associated with the erupting deciduous or permanent teeth in children. This cyst has often been termed as 'eruption cyst' or 'eruption hematoma'.

It is essentially a dilation of the normal tooth caused by accumulation of tissue fluid or blood. Clinically, the lesion appears as a circumscribed, fluctuant, often translucent swelling of the alveolar ridge over the site of eruption of the tooth. When the circumscribed cystic cavity contains blood the swelling appears purple or, deep blue, hence, it is termed as 'eruption hematoma'.

Radiographically expansion of the normal follicular space of erupting tooth crown (Fig. 4.5). In some cases there is saucer shaped excavation of bone projecting very slightly into the cavity.

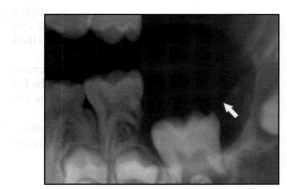

Fig. 4.5: Eruption cyst showing expansion of follicular space (*Courtesy:* Dr Ashok L, Professor and Head, Oral Medicine and Radiology, Bapuji Dental College and Hospital Davangere, Karnataka)

ODONTOGENIC KERATOCYST

The keratocyst was probably first described by Mikulicz in 1876. According to Pindborg's and Hansen the designation keratocyst was used to described any jaw cyst exhibiting keratinization in their lining which may occur in follicular, residual and very rarely in a radicular cyst.

OKC is not a clinical diagnosis but a designation for a group of cysts of possibly diverse origins which have a number of highly characteristic microscopic and clinical features in common with highest recurrences rate of any of the odontogenic cyst.

It is originated from dental lamina which still possesses marked growth potential or alternatively from proliferation of basal cells as 'basal cell hamartias'. The epithelium of the odontogenic keratocyst has been shown to be far more active than most odontogenic cysts as judged by their greater mitotic activity.

It is more common in mandible with a greater incidence at the angle and extending for varying distance into the ascending ramus and forward into the body. Asymptomatic unless they become secondarily infected, in which case patient complains of pain, soft tissue swelling and drainage (Fig. 4.6). Occasionally, they experience paraesthesia of the lower lip. Teeth may be displaced, if OKC expands through cancellous bone and the body of the mandible. The lesion can lead to pathologic fracture. Multiple odontogenic keratocyst are found in following syndromes: Gorlin- Goltz syndrome, Marfan's syndrome, Ehler's Danlos syndrome and Noonan's syndrome.

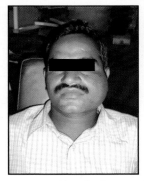

Fig. 4.6: OKC involving a ramus. Note the huge swelling on the ramus on left side (*Courtesy:* Dr Tapasya Karamore, Lecturer, Oral Medicine and Radiology, VSPM Dental College and Research Center, Nagpur, India)

Radiologically undulating borders, cloudy interior appearances suggestive of multilocularity. Size varies and may be 5 cm or more in diameter. Maxillary lesions are smaller and rounder than those in the mandible. Shape of cyst is usually oval extending along the body of the mandible with little mediolateral expansion (Fig. 4.7). Margins are hyperostotic and tooth displacement is seen. Majority of lesions are unilocular with smooth borders but some unilocular lesions are large with irregular borders. Radiolucency is usually hazy due to keratin filled cavity and it is surrounded by thin sclerotic rim due to reactive osteocytes.

It can expand and perforate the buccal and lingual cortical plates of bone and involve the adjacent soft tissue

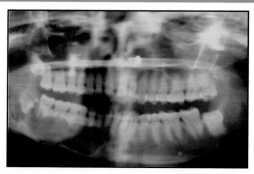

Fig. 4.7: Odontogenic keratocyst showing destruction in anteroposterior direction in the right side of mandible

(Fig. 4.8). Downward displacement of the inferior alveolar canal and resorption of the lower cortical plate of the mandible may be seen. As the keratocyst enlarges it may produce deflection of unerupted teeth mostly in the region of the angle of the mandible and occasionally, on the ascending ramus (Fig. 4.9) and towards the orbital floor and in some cases root resorption is also seen.

Radiologically, it may be envelopment type (embraces an adjacent unerupted tooth), replacement (forms in the place of normal teeth, extraneous (those in the ascending ramus away from the teeth), (Fig. 4.9) collateral (those adjacent to the root of teeth which are indistinguishable from the lateral periodontal cyst).

It is managed by enucleation of entire cyst with vigorous curettage of the cystic wall.

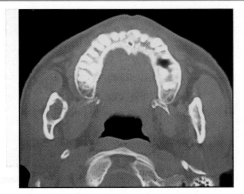

Fig. 4.8: 3D CT picture of odontogenic keratocyst on left side of mandible. (*Courtesy:* E. Ariji)

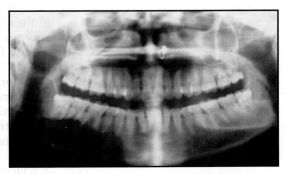

Fig. 4.9: Extraneous type of odontogenic keratocyst showing lesion in the ramus

PRIMORDIAL CYST

It is one of the less common types of odontogenic cysts.

It originates when cystic changes take place in the stellate reticulum of the tooth germ before any calcified enamel or dentin has been formed. So it is found in place of a tooth rather than directly associated with it.

It has a tendency to painlessly enlarge and slowly replace large portions of cancellous bone before expansion of the cortical plate by way of which it reveals its presence. Pain which is associated with a large cyst is caused by infection that may follow the perforation of the expanded cortical plate.

Radiologically cyst like radiolucency that is well-defined and have hyperostotic borders (Fig. 4.10). It may be unilocular or have a scalloped outline that gives it a multilocular appearance.

Surgical enucleation should be done.

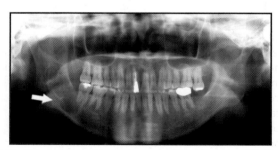

Fig. 4.10: Primordial cyst involving mandible (*Courtesy:* Eiichiro Ariji, Professor and Head, Department of Oral and Maxillofacial Radiology, Acihi-Gakuin University School of Dentistry, Nagoya, Japan)

LATERAL PERIODONTAL CYST

The lateral periodontal cyst is uncommon but a well recognized type of developmental odontogenic cyst. The designation lateral periodontal cyst is confined to that cyst, which occurs as a result of inflammatory etiology and the diagnosis of collateral keratocyst has been excluded on clinical and histological ground.

It can originated from dentigerious cyst developing along the lateral surface of the crown, from proliferation of cell rests of Malassez in the periodontal ligament, primordial cyst of a supernumerary tooth germ, from proliferation and cystic transformation of rests of dental lamina.

It can be inflammatory (pocket content may irritate and stimulate rest of malassez) developmental (associated with developing tooth germ).

Gingival swelling may occur on the facial aspect and in these types of cases; it must be differentiated from the gingival cyst. In gingival cyst the overlying mucosa is blue but in lateral periodontal cyst the overlying mucosa appears normal. The associated tooth is vital. If the cyst becomes infected, it may resemble a lateral periodontal abscess.

Radiologically, the intra-bony lateral periodontal cyst is seen as a round or ovoid well-defined radiolucency with hyperostotic borders (Fig. 4.11). It is found between the cervical margins and the apex of adjacent root surfaces and may or may not be in contact with root surfaces.

The lateral periodontal cyst must be surgically removed.

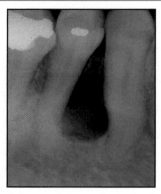

Fig. 4.11: Radiolucency between the roots of premolar and the canine suggesting lateral periodontal cyst

GINGIVAL CYST OF ADULT

It is an uncommon cyst occurring either on free or attached gingiva. It is caused by degenerative changes in proliferating epithelial tissue, remnants of dental lamina, enamel organ or epithelial islands of periodontal membrane, traumatic implantation of epithelium and arises from post-functional rests of dental lamina.

It is slowly enlarging, painless swelling, usually less than 1 cm in diameter and may occur in attached gingiva or the interdental papilla. The surface may be smooth and the color may appear as that of normal gingiva or bluish (Fig. 4.12) and may appear red when it is blood filled as a result of recent trauma. The lesions are soft and fluctuant and

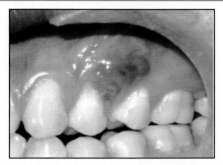

Fig. 4.12: Gingival cyst in the premolar region which is bluish in color (*Courtesy:* Dr Abhishek Soni, Lecturer, Periodontology, VSPM Dental College and Research Centre, Nagpur, India)

adjacent teeth are usually vital during surgical exploration. Slight erosion on the surface of the bone may be observed without extension into the periodontium.

Radiologically there may be no radiological changes or only a faint round shadow indicative of superficial bone erosion (Fig. 4.13).

Surgical excision of the lesion in adults is usually recommended and the lesion does not tend to recur.

CALCIFYING EPITHELIUM ODONTOGENIC CYST

It is also called as 'keratinizing and calcifying odontogenic cyst' and 'Gorlin's cyst' as it was first described by Gorlin in 1962. The lesion is unusual in that it has some features suggestive of cyst but also has many characteristic of a solid

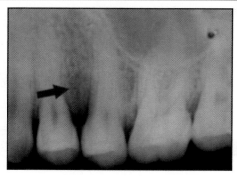

Fig. 4.13: Note the superficial erosion seen in gingival cyst (*Courtesy:* Dr Abhishek Soni, Lecturer, Periodontology, VSPM Dental College and Research Centre, Nagpur, India)

neoplasm. Central calcifying odontogenic cyst is also known as intra-osseous odontogenic cyst.

It is slow growing, painless, non-tender swelling of the jaws. Occasionally some patients may complain of pain. In some cases, cortical plate over the expanding lesion may be destroyed and cystic mass may be palpable. Adjacent teeth may be displaced.

Radiologically, the central lesion may appear as a cyst like radiolucency with variable margins which may be quite smooth with a well-defined outline or irregular in shape with poorly defined borders (Fig. 4.14). Roots of adjacent teeth may resorb. It may contain small foci of calcified material that are only microscopically apparent.

Enucleation and curettage should be done.

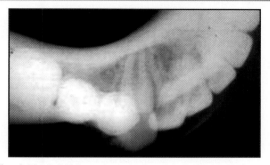

Fig. 4.14: Calcifying odontogenic cyst showing calcification

RADICULAR CYST

It is also called as 'apical periodontal cyst', 'periapical cyst', or 'dental root end cyst'. It is a common sequel in progressive changes associated with bacterial invasion and death of the dental pulp. It most commonly occurs at the apices of teeth.

Periradicular inflammatory changes cause the epithelium to proliferate. As the epithelium grows into a mass of cells, the center losses the source of nutrition from the periapical tissue. These changes produce necrosis in the center and a cavity is formed and cyst is created.

It represents an asymptomatic phase in periapical inflammatory process following death of the dental pulp. It is associated with non vital tooth. It rarely causes non tender expansion of the overlying cortical bone. Swelling may be bony hard or crepitations may be present as bone is thinned

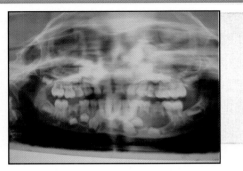

Fig. 4.15: Radicular cyst in association with deciduous first molar on left side (crop image)

or it may be rubbery or fluctuate, if the bone is completely destroyed.

Radiologically, it appears as a rounded or pear shaped radiolucency at the apex of nonsensitive tooth or with nonvital tooth (Fig. 4.15). Radiolucency is more than 1.5 cm in diameter but usually less than 3 cm in diameter (Fig. 4.16). It has got well-defined outline with thin hyperostotic borders. Margins are smooth, corticated and the cortex is usually well-defined, continuous. Radicular cysts of long duration may cause resorption of roots.

It is managed by root canal treatment; extraction of offending tooth, in some large cyst enucleation is done.

RESIDUAL CYST

It is a cyst that either remained as such in the jaw when it's associated tooth was removed or was formed in residual

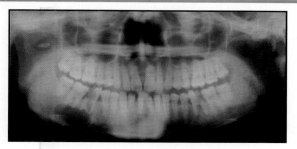

Fig. 4.16: Radicular cyst associated with right first molar which is carious

epithelium of cell rests from a periodontal ligament of the lost tooth. Low grade inflammation of parent cyst might predispose formation of residual cyst.

It is asymptomatic with a previous history of pain in the tooth. It is seldom more than 5 to 10 mm in diameter.

Radiologically pre-extraction radiographs show tooth with an evidence of deep caries or fracture adequate for pulp involvement and/or an associated cyst. It is round or ovoid radiolucency that is usually well circumscribed (Fig. 4.17). Thin radiopaque margins are common with unilocular appearance although the infected cyst will not have such well-defined margins.

Enucleation is done.

PARADENTAL CYST

It was first described by Craig in 1976. It is a cyst of inflammatory origin occurring on the lateral aspect of the

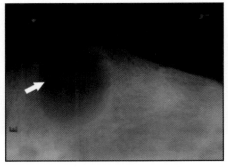

Fig. 4.17: Residual cyst seen as well-defined radiolucency side (*Courtesy:* Dr Tapasya Karamore, Lecturer, Oral Medicine and Radiology, VSPM Dental College and Research Center, Nagpur, India)

root of partially erupted mandibular third molar with an associated history of pericornitis.

It is originated from cell rests of malassez or from the reduced enamel epithelium.

Radiologically there is well demarcated radiolucency occurring distal to the partially erupted tooth (Fig. 4.18) but there was often buccal superimposition. The radiolucency sometimes extends apically but an intact periodontal ligament space provided the evidence that the lesion did not originates at the apex.

The lesion is treated by surgical enucleation.

MANDIBULAR BUCCAL INFECTED CYST

It is an inflammatory cyst occurring on the buccal surface of mandibular molars in young children.

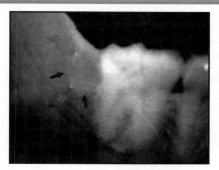

Fig. 4.18: Paradental cyst seen associated with the third molar

There may be discomfort, pain, tenderness and rarely suppuration. Swelling particularly, if inflamed, is the clinical feature most likely to induce the patient to seek advice. Facial swelling may follow and this may be inflamed. The associated tooth is usually tilted, so that the apices are adjacent to the lingual cortex, a feature which is demonstrable in occlusal radiographs. The cyst extension in buccal direction is variable, but frequently the outer bony cortex is lost.

With involvement of the periosteum new bone may be laid down either as a single linear band or laminated, if there two or more layers (Fig. 4.19). Sometimes, the new bone may be homogeneous. The cysts will appear on the buccal aspects of the affected molars. The inferior margins of the cyst are concave and rarely, the cyst may extend to the inferior border of the mandible but not leading to any external deformity.

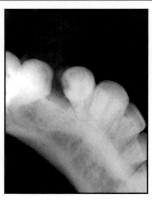

Fig. 4.19: Mandibular buccal infected cyst showing
new bone formation on buccal side

It is generally agreed that enucleation of the cyst without
removal of the associated tooth is the treatment of choice.

NASOPALATINE CYST

It is also called as 'nasopalatine duct cyst', 'incisive canal
cyst', 'median anterior maxillary cyst' or 'vestigial cyst'. It is
the most common non-odontogenic cyst in the oral cavity.

It is developmental in origin and arises in the incisive
canal when embryonic epithelial remnants of the
nasopalatine duct undergo proliferation and cystic
transformation.

There is a small well-defined swelling just posterior to
the palatine papilla. Sometime, it may become infected,

producing pain. Patients complain of salty taste in mouth produced by small sinus or remnant of nasopalatine duct that permits cystic fluid to drain into oral cavity. Burning sensation and numbness may be experience due to pressure on the nasopalatine nerve. Sometimes cystic fluid may drain and patient reports a salty taste.

Deeper cysts are covered by normal mucosa, unless it is ulcerated. If cyst expands, it may penetrate the labial plate and produce a swelling below the maxillary labial frenum.

Radiologically cyst like radiolucency superimposed with the apices of the central incisors. Image of radiopaque anterior nasal spine may superimpose over the dark cystic cavity giving it a heart shape or shape of inverted tear drop. Cyst in canal cavity also erodes the bone posterior to the canal and creates impression of midpalatal cyst. In many cases, cyst is situated symmetrically in the midline (Fig. 4.20). It may be rounded, oval or irregularly shaped. Divergence of central incisor roots and external root resorption is common.

Its removal is not indicated unless there are clinical symptoms.

GLOBULOMAXILLARY CYST

It is also called as 'intra-alveolar cyst'. It occurs in globulomaxillary area. It was considered to be an inclusion or developmental cyst that arises from entrapped non-odontogenic epithelium in globulomaxillary suture which occurs at the junction of globular portion of the medial nasal process and maxillary process.

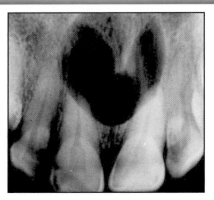

Fig. 4.20: Incisive canal cyst note heart shaped radiolucency

It is asymptomatic and is discovered during routine radiographical examination. If cyst becomes infected, patient may complain of local discomfort or pain in that area. As it enlarges, it expands the buccal cortical plate between maxillary lateral incisors and canines. It may diverge the roots of two teeth and their crown may rotate causing the contact point to move incisally. Adjacent teeth are usually vital. If cortical plate is eroded then fluctuant swelling develops. Palpation will produce crepitus.

Radiologically, it appears as pear-shaped or tear-shaped radiolucency between roots of maxillary lateral incisors and canines (Fig. 4.21). Small end of the pear is directed toward the crest of alveolar ridge. The upper border may invaginate the floor of the nasal fossa or the antrum. The size is variable

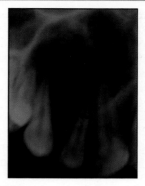

Fig. 4.21: Pear shaped radiolucency in between the lateral incisor and the canine

and may reach the maximum level of diameter of 3-4 cm. It may cause divergence of the roots adjacent teeth. Displacement of the teeth is common. It is well-defined and lamina dura of the adjacent teeth are usually intact. There may be root resorption.

Enucleation should be done.

TRAUMATIC BONE CYST

It is also known as 'solitary bone cyst', 'hemorrhagic bone cyst', 'extravasation cyst', 'simple bone cyst', 'unicameral cyst' and 'idiopathic bone cavity'. The traumatic bone cyst is a misnomer, since these intra-bony cavities are not lined by epithelium. It results from trauma induced intra-medullary hematoma with subsequently result in bone resorption and cavitations during hematoma resolution.

It is asymptomatic in most cases but occasionally, there may be evidence of pain and tenderness. Cortical swelling or slight tooth movement are not the usual finding and the teeth are vital. Needle aspiration is actually unproductive and if it is productive it contains either a small amount of straw colored fluid shed off necrotic blood clot and fragment of fibrous connective tissue.

Radiologically it appears as a radiolucent lesion with a spectrum of well-defined to moderately defined borders. Most cases are unilocular with a fairly regular border (Fig. 4.22). There is evidence of hyperostotic borders around the entire lesion but occasionally such border is lacking. Most characteristic radiographic feature of this cyst is scalloped superior or occlusal margins where it extends between the roots of the teeth.

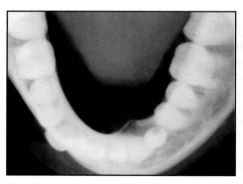

Fig. 4.22: Traumatic bone cyst showing hyperostotic border

ANEURYSMAL BONE CYST

It is an uncommon hemorrhagic lesion of the bone which is rarely seen in the jaw. It is most often categorized as to be a tumor like reactive lesion of bone. The name of this entity is misleading, in that, it does not contain vascular aneurysms and it is not a true bony cyst.

It represents an exaggerated localized proliferative response of the vascular tissue.

Persistent local alteration in hemodynamics leads to increased venous pressure and development of dilated and engorged vessels in transformed bone area. Resorption of bone occurs, to which giant cells are related and this is replaced by connective tissue, osteoid and new bone.

Aneurysmal cyst of the jaw produces a firm swelling which may be painful and tender on motion. Usually, there is tilting or bodily displacement of teeth in the affected areas. Excessive bleeding may occur.

Radiologically, it is an expansile osteolytic process within the affected bone and is projected as a definite radiolucency. Fine septa are seen crossing through the lesion in a random pattern. The term 'soap bubble' may be applied to describe an occasional multilocular radiographic appearance.

Surgical curettage or partial resections are the primary forms of treatment for aneurysmal bone cyst.

DERMOID AND EPIDERMOID CYST

It may occur as developmental anomalies and about 1 to 2 percent occurs in oral cavity. The lumen of simple cyst filled with cyst fluid or keratin and no other specialized structure, is called as 'epidermoid cyst'. If lumen contains sebaceous material as well as keratin then it is called as 'dermoid cyst'. If lumen contains elements such as bone, muscle or teeth from various germinal layer is called as 'teratoma'.

Swelling is slow and painless. It may interfere with breathing, speaking, closing the mouth and eating. The size may vary up to several centimeters in diameter (Fig. 4.23). Transillumination test is usually negative. Fluctuation test is generally positive.

Radiologically in some cases, if you want to see the extent of the cyst, then we have to remove some content of the cyst to enable introduction of an opaque substance such as lipiodol, which is chemical combination of iodine and

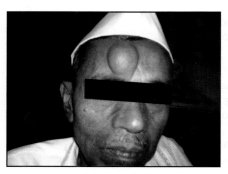

Fig. 4.23: Dermoid cyst seen on the forehead which is well-defined

poppyseed oil. After this, radiograph is made from every position necessary to enable opaque material find its way by gravity to each portion of the cyst.

Surgical excision is the treatment of choice.

JAW CYST-BASAL CELL NEVUS-BIFID RIB SYNDROME

It is also called as 'nevoid basal cell carcinoma', 'Gorlin's and Goltz's syndrome'. It is transmitted as autosomal dominant trait with poor degree of penetrance and variable expressivity.

Cutaneous Anomalies

Basal cell carcinoma, dermal cyst and tumors, palmar pitting, palmar and plantar keratosis and dermal calcinosis. Skin lesions are small, flattened, flesh colored or brownish papules occurring anywhere in the body, but are prominent on the face and trunk.

Skeletal Abnormalities

Rib anomalies and brachymetacarpalism, bifid rib, agenesis, deformity and synostosis of rib; kyphoscoliosis, vertebral fusion, polydactyly and shortening of metacarpals.

Ophthalmologic Abnormalities

Hypertelorism with wide nasal bridge, dystopia canthorum, congenital blindness and internal strabismus.

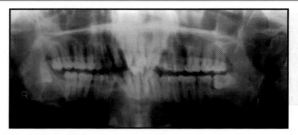

Fig. 4.24: Multiple OKC seen in case of jaw cyst basal cell Nevus syndrome (*Courtesy:* Dr Ashok L, Professor and Head, Department of Oral Medicine and Radiology, Bapuji Dental College and Hospital, Davanagere, India)

Neurological Anomalies

Mental retardation, calcification of falx cerebri and other parts of dura, agenesis of corpus callosum, congenital hydrocephalus and occurrence of medulloblastomas.

Sexual Abnormalities

Hypogonadism in males and ovarian tumors.

Orally jaw lesions appear as multiple odontogenic keratocysts usually appearing in multiple quadrants. Mild mandibular prognathism.

Radiologically jaw cysts appear as a multiple cyst like radiolucency of variable size varying from few millimeters to several centimeters (Fig. 4.24). They occur most frequently in premolar-molar region. Radiopaque lines of calcified falx cerebri are prominent on PA projection.

It is managed by complete enucleation of the lesion should be done. Periodic examination.

Odontogenic Tumor

ADENOMATOID ODONTOGENIC TUMOR

It is also called as 'Adenoameloblastoma' or 'ameloblastic adenomatoid tumor'. It is tumor of odontogenic epithelium with a duct like structure and varying degrees of inductive changes in the connective tissue.

It commonly presented as an area of swelling over an unerupted tooth which is asymptomatic (Fig. 5.1). Some times it may expand cortical bone but is not invasive. It is frequently associated with an unerupted tooth in which the epithelial proliferation is confined within a connective tissue capsule that is attached to the tooth in manner similar to the attachment of a dentigerous cyst. When the tumor occurs independently of unerupted teeth it is often encapsulated. The tumor causes expansion of bone and fluctuation may be elicited.

Radiologically well-demarcated mixed radiolucent or opaque lesion site - tumor surrounds the entire tooth, most often canine in the maxilla (Fig. 5.2). Radiolucency usually extends apically beyond the cementoenamel junction. It may or may not be well circumscribed.

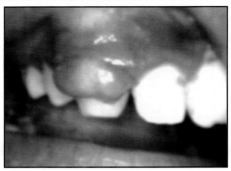

Fig. 5.1: Adenomatoid tumor presenting as a swelling in the maxillary anterior region (*Courtesy:* Dr Tapasya Karamore, Lecturer Department of Oral Medicine and Radiology, VSPM Dental College and Research Centre, Nagpur, India)

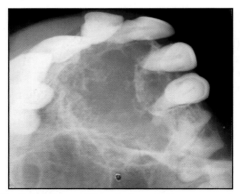

Fig. 5.2: Adenomatoid odontogenic tumor presented as radiolucency in anterior maxillary region

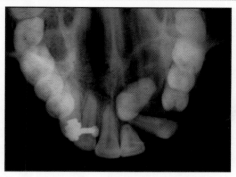

Fig. 5.3: AOT presenting as small pebbles appearance (*Courtesy:* Dr Mody, Professor and Head, Oral Medicine and Radiology, GDCH, Nagpur)

Unilocular radiolucency but may contain faint to dense radiopaque foci which may be seen peripherally as the lesion matures. Dense cluster of radiopacities appear as 'small pebbles' (Fig. 5.3).

Separation of roots or displacement of a adjacent tooth occurs frequently. There is also cortical expansion and root resorption.

Conservative surgical excision and curettage can be effective.

AMELOBLASTIC FIBROMA

It is also called as 'fibrous adamantinoma', 'soft odontoma', 'soft mixed odontoma', 'granular cell ameloblastic fibroma' and 'fibroadamanblastoma'. It is characterized by simultaneous proliferation of both epithelial and mesenchymal tissue without formation of enamel and dentin.

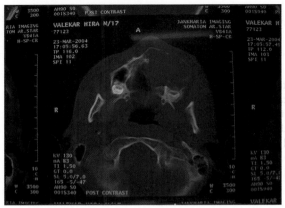

Fig. 5.4: Ameloblastic fibroma showing expansion of bone (*Courtesy:* Dr Bhaskar Patle, Lecturer, Oral Medicine and Radiology, SPDC, Wardha, India)

It is painless and expands slowly. There is bulging of the cortical plates rather than erosion through them. There is also migration of involved teeth. It enlarges by gradual expansion so that the periphery of bone often remains smooth. It is associated with unerupted teeth.

Radiologically it may present with cyst like area of bone destruction (Fig. 5.4) or there may wide area of bone destruction. As it is usually associated with an impacted tooth, it appears as pericoronal radiolucency. It develops in premolarmolar area of the mandible. Margin are well defined often with sclerotic borders.

Curettage can be done which has successful results in many cases.

CALCIFYING EPITHELIAL ODONTOGENIC TUMOR

It is also called as 'Pindborg tumor' or 'calcifying amelo-blastoma'. It arises from the reduced enamel epithelium or dental epithelium.

It is asymptomatic and only presenting symptom is a painless swelling (Fig. 5.5). In rare cases, there is associated mild paresthesia. Cortical expansion occurs. Palpation will show hard tumor with well defined or diffuse border. It is locally invasive with a high recurrence rate.

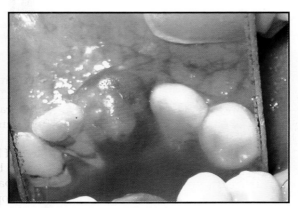

Fig. 5.5: Calcifying epithelial odontogenic cyst (*Courtesy:* Dr Abhishek Soni, Lecturer, Periodontia, VSPM Dental College and Research Center, Nagpur, India)

Radiologically it may be totally radiolucent to mostly radiopaque area around the crown of unerupted teeth. The radiopacity is produced by mineralization of amorphous proteinaceous material generated by the tumor cells rather than the disorganized formation of dental tissue. Margin may or may not be well demarcated from the surrounding normal tissue. There may be a combined pattern of radiolucency and radiopacities with many small, irregular bony trabeculae traversing the radiolucent area in many directions producing a multilocular or honey comb pattern.

Later, it reveals a unilocular or a multilocular cystic lesion with numerous scattered radiopaque foci of varying sizes and density which gives it an appearance as that of 'driven snow' (Fig. 5.6).

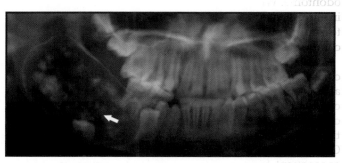

Fig. 5.6: CEOT driven snow appearance (*Courtesy:* Dr Mody, Professor and Head, Oral Medicine and Radiology, GDCH, Nagpur, India)

ODONTOMA

It is a hamartoma of odontogenic origin in which both epithelial and mesenchymal cells exhibit complete differentiation with enamel and dentin laid down in abnormal position.

It can be complex or compound type, both the epithelial and mesenchymal cells exhibit complete differentiation with the result that functional ameloblasts and odontoblasts form enamel and dentin. Lesion is composed of more than one type of tissue, for this reason it is called as composite odontome. In some composite odontomes, the enamel and dentin are laid down in such a fashion that the structure bears a considerable anatomical resemblance to that of normal teeth except they are often smaller than the typical teeth, which have been termed as compound composite odontome. When calcified dental tissue are simply arranged in a irregular mass bearing no morphological similarity even to rudimentary tooth then that form is called as complex composite odontome.

Compound occurs in incisor, canine area of maxilla and complex occurs in mandibular 1st and 2nd molar area. It is also occur in inferior border of the mandible, ramus and condylar region. Compound odontoma is between 1 to 3 cms in diameter. It usually remains small and diameter of the mass only occasionally increases than that of the tooth. Occasionally, it may produce expansion of bone with consequent facial asymmetry. Sometime cyst develops in relation with a complex odontome and compound odontome, but it is very rare.

Radiologically it appears as an irregular mass of calcified material surrounded by narrow radiolucent bands with a small outer periphery. Compound type shows number of teeth like structures in the region of the canine (Fig. 5.7). There is cluster of small shapeless dense masses of solid tissue having equal or more density, depending on the size of the mass. There may be many masses each of which has own dark line surrounding it. If a large number of teeth are present, the radiopaque mass is surrounded by a radiolucent line that represents the pericoronal space of the unerupted teeth.

Complex composite odontoma appears as a dense radiopaque object sometimes lying in clear space. Density is greater than that of bone and to greater than or equal to the

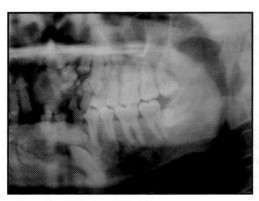

Fig. 5.7: Compound odontome (*Courtesy:* Dr Amit Parate, Lecturer, Oral Medicine and Radiology, GDCH, Nagpur, India)

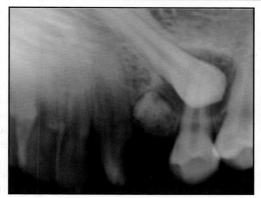

Fig. 5.8: Cystic complex odontome surrounded by dark shadow

teeth. It shows a well defined radiolucency containing irregular masses of calcified tissue (Fig. 5.8). It is associated with unerupted teeth.

AMELOBLASTOMA

First detailed description of ameloblastoma was given by 'Falkson' in 1879. It is an aggressive tumor that appears to be arising from remnants of dental lamina or dental organs. It is the most common epithelial tumor producing minimal inductive changes.

It is a benign but locally invasive polymorphic neoplasm consisting of proliferating odontogenic epithelium.

Neoplasm is frequently preceded by extraction of teeth, cystectomy and some other traumatic episodes. It begins as

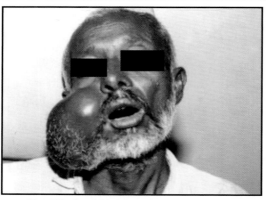

Fig. 5.9: Ameloblastoma presenting as huge swelling and expansion of the jaw

a central lesion of the bone which is slowly destructive but tends to expand bone rather than perforating it. Patient notices a gradually increasing facial asymmetry (Fig. 5.9). Teeth in involved region are displaced and become mobile. Pain and paresthesia may occur, if the lesion is pressing upon a nerve or is secondarily infected. In later stages, the lesion may show ovoid and fusiform enlargement that is hard but non tender (Fig. 5.10). As tumor enlarges palpation may elicit a hard sensation or crepitus. Surrounding bone may become so thin that fluctuation and 'egg shell crackling' may be elicited. If it is left untreated for many years the expansion may be extremely disfiguring, fungating and ulcerative type of growth characteristic of that of carcinoma can be seen.

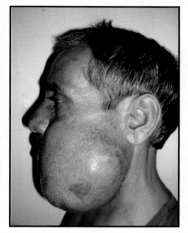

Fig. 5.10: Ameloblastoma on left side at the angle of mandible appearing as a huge swelling (*Courtesy:* Dr Bhaskar Patle, Lecturer, Oral Medicine and Radiology, SPDC, Wardha, India)

Radiologically in early stages, there is area of bone destruction which is well defined and is indicative of slow growth with hyperostotic borders. Outline is smooth, scalloped, well defined and well corticated. The walls of the cavity are coarse. In some cases the margins of the tumor are lobulated. Usually it is multilocular but may be unilocular.

There is presence of septa in the lesion. In some cases, number and arrangement of septa may give the area a 'honeycomb appearance' (Fig. 5.11) (numerous small compartments) or a 'soap bubble appearance' (larger compartments).

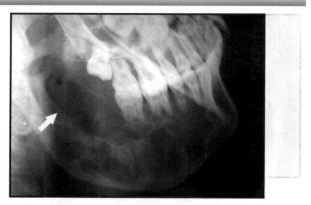

Fig. 5.11: Honeycomb appearance of ameloblastoma (*Courtesy:* Dr Mody, Professor and Head, Oral Medicine and Radiology, GDCH, Nagpur India)

In advanced stages, perforated cortical plate may contribute to a multilocular appearance.

The jaws are likely to be enlarged, depending on the over all size of the tumor (Fig. 5.12). Extensive root resorption may occur. Thickening of membrane, cloudiness and destruction of walls are the finding when the sinus is involved. Expansion and thinning of cortical plate occurs leaving thin 'egg shell of bone'. Perforation of bone is a late feature.

It is managed by curettage, intraoral block excision, extraoral en bloc resection, and peripheral osteotomy.

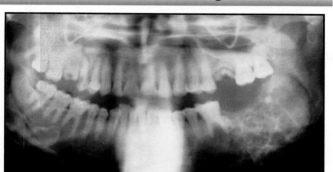

Fig. 5.12: Ameloblastoma on left side of mandible which involve ramus also

SQUAMOUS ODONTOGENIC TUMOR

It is well differentiated odontogenic tumor composed of islands or sheets of squamous epithelium that lack recognizable features of enamel organ differentiation.

It arises from the rests of malassez, although hamartomatous epithelial transformation is also found.

It is usually asymptomatic but there may be mobility of the involved teeth, pain, tenderness to percussion and occasionally abnormal sensation.

Radiologically it occurs usually in association with the cervical portion of the tooth. It is well circumscribed radiolucent area which presents as a semi-circular or roughly triangular area (Fig. 5.13). Border may or may not be sclerotic.

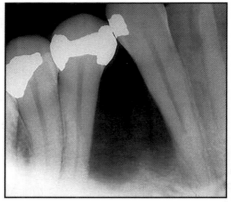

Fig. 5.13: Squamous odontogenic tumor seen as semicircular radiolucency

Conservative enucleation and curettage is usually curative with a low recurrence rate.

ODONTOGENIC MYXOMA

It is also called as 'odontogenic fibro-myxoma', 'myxofibroma'. It is a rare non-invasive neoplasm that arises from the dental papilla, follicular mesenchyme and periodontal ligament.

It is associated with congenitally missing teeth. The growth rate is slow and pain is variable. There is a hard swelling which may be sometime large enough to produce facial asymmetry. Sometimes it perforates the cortical plate producing a bosselated surface (several small nodules on the surface). It may appear as fusiform swelling that may be hard and or may be covered by a layer of bone of only egg shell.

Radiologically it may be either unilocular or multilocular. It may be mixed radiopaque-radiolucent lesion. Compartments tend to be angular. They may be separated by straight septa that form square, rectangular or triangular spaces. The central portion is transversed by fine trabeculation. It is usually well defined but sometimes it may be poorly defined. It may be scalloped between the roots of adjacent teeth.

Locules are small and uniform with typical honeycomb appearance or strings of tennis racket (Fig. 5.14).

Exceptionally, fine septa cross the radiolucent area producing a soap bubble appearance.

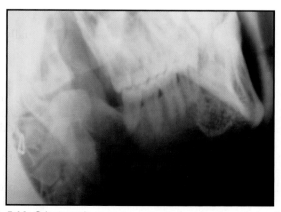

Fig. 5.14: Odontogenic myxoma presented as tennis racket pattern

Tumors may be difficult to enucleate due to their loose consistency, therefore surgical excision is indicated.

PERIPHERAL ODONTOGENIC FIBROMA

It is also called as 'peripheral ossifying fibroma', 'peripheral ameloblastic fibro-dentinoma', 'calcifying fibrous epulis' peripheral fibroma with calcification. It consists of fibrous tissue containing nests of odontogenic epithelium and calcified material that resembles cementum.

It involves periodontal ligament superficially.

It is usually asymptomatic. It is slow growing, often present for a number of years. Some lesions grow large enough to cause facial asymmetry. They are solid and firmly attached to the gingival mass, (Fig. 5.15) sometimes arise

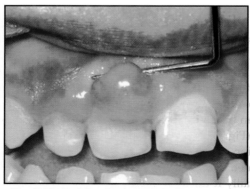

Fig. 5.15: Peripheral odontogenic fibroma in the region of maxilla in free gingival margin

between teeth and sometimes displaced the teeth. It is well demarcated mass of tissue on the gingiva with a sessile or pedunculated base (Fig. 5.15). Early lesions are soft, quite vascular and red and bleed readily. More mature lesions are firm fibrous and pale pink.

Radiologically on rare occasions there may be superficial erosion of bone.

Simple surgical excision.

CENTRAL ODONTOGENIC FIBROMA

It is a lesion around the crown of an unerupted tooth resembling a small dentigerous cyst. But some say that it is a hyperplastic dental follicle and not an odontogenic tumor. It may occur centrally or in the periphery. Peripheral variant clinically mimics fibroma.

It is generally asymptomatic except for the swelling of the jaws. It may cause localized bony expansion or loosening of teeth.

Radiologically it produces an expansile radiolucency similar to that of ameloblastoma. It is often associated with apices of erupted teeth. Margins are well defined and sclerotic. It can be unilocular but larger lesions tend to be multilocular (Fig. 5.16). Larger lesions cause root divergence and resorption.

Treated with enucleation and curettage. Surgical excision and usually it does not recur.

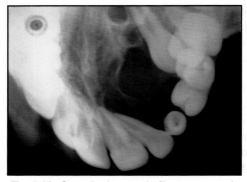

Fig. 5.16: Central odontogenic fibroma presenting
as multilocular radiolucency with root divergence

PERIAPICAL CEMENTAL DYSPLASIA

It is also called as 'fibrocementoma', 'sclerosing cementum',
'periapical osteofibrosis', 'periapical fibrosarcoma'. It is a
reactive fibro-osseous lesion derived from the odontogenic
cells in the periodontal ligament. It is located at the apex of
the teeth.

It is caused by local factors (trauma, chronic irritation),
hormone, nutritional deficiency, metabolic disturbances,
past history of syphilis, endocrinal imbalance and anomalous development.

It is seen only in female. Involved teeth are vital with no
history of pain or sensitivity. Occasional lesions localize
near the mental foramen and impinge on the mental nerve
and produce pain, paresthesia or even anesthesia. Hypercementosis is usually associated with it. It rarely enlarges.

Radiologically margin are well defined. A radiolucent border of varying width, surrounded by band of sclerotic bone is seen. Sclerotic bone represents immediate reaction of surrounding bone.

Stage I: Radiolucent (Fibrous)

Since there is loss of bony substance and replacement by connective tissue, the lesions appear radiolucent. There is formation of a circumscribed area of periapical fibrosis accompanied by localized bone destruction (Fig. 5.17). The margins of the radiolucent area vary in different lesion; some

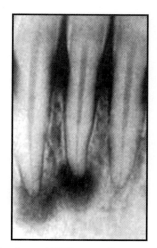

Fig. 5.17: Early stage of PCD presenting as radiolucent lesion

are well defined but not corticated and others are poorly defined or well defined at one portion of the lesion and ill defined elsewhere. Lamina dura around the tooth is lost.

Stage II: Mixed Stage

Margins of the opacity are usually sharp but sometimes it can be ill defined and irregular. Minute radiopacities are seen within the radiolucent periapical area due to either bone or cementum formation (Fig. 5.18). It is called as cementoblastic stage. Small radiopacities may coalesce. It has round, oval or irregular shape.

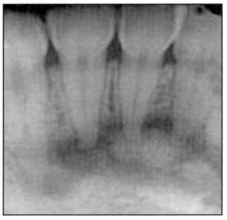

Fig. 5.18: Mixed stage of PCD showing radiopacity as well radiolucency

Stage III: Radiopaque

There is complete opacification. It appears as a well defined radiopacity usually bordered by a radiolucent capsule separating it from the adjacent bone (Fig. 5.19). Margins may vary from well defined to poorly define. Lamina dura of adjacent teeth may be discontinuous in the area of lesion. Hypercementosis is produced in some cases which can be seen at the apex.

Surgical enucleation is indicated for larger lesions which have caused expansion of the cortical plates or when the clinician is unsure of the working diagnosis.

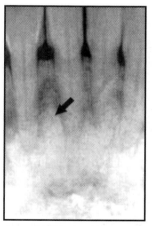

Fig. 5.19: Mature stage of PCD showing complete radiopaque lesion

BENIGN CEMENTOBLASTOMA

It is also called as 'true Cementoma'. There is large bulbous mass of cementum or cementum like tissue on roots of teeth. It is rare benign odontogenic neoplasm which arises from the cementoblast.

It is derived from periodontal ligament.

Pain may be there but it may be associated to carious teeth rather than the disease itself. Involved tooth is vital and the lesion is slow growing and it may cause expansion of the jaw (Fig. 5.20). In some cases it may displace the involved tooth.

Radiologically well defined radiopacities usually attached to the roots of premolars and molars surrounded

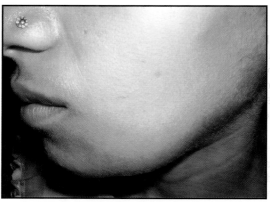

Fig. 5.20: Benign cementoblastoma seen as swelling extraorally

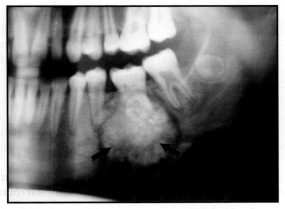

Fig. 5.21: Cementoblastoma seen as well defined radiopaque mass surrounded by a radiolucent halo

at the border by a radiolucent halo are seen (Fig. 5.21). They are mixed radiolucent-radiopaque lesion that may be amorphous or may have wheel like spoke pattern. Density of cementum obscures the outline of the enveloped root. Occlusal radiograph will demonstrate its expansive nature.

Excision with extraction of the associated tooth.

AMELOBLASTIC FIBRO-ODONTOMA

The name is applied to an odontogenic lesion that exhibits mixed epithelial-mesenchymal proliferation and both mature and immature areas.

The most common presenting complaint is swelling and failure of tooth eruption. The maxillary tumor if large

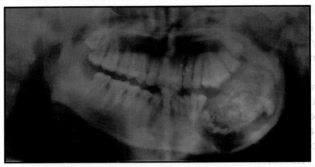

Fig. 5.22: Ameloblastic fibro-odontoma presented as an expansile lesion in the mandible (*Courtesy:* Dr Amit Parate, Lecturer, Oral Medicine and Radiology, GDCH, Nagpur, India)

interferes with nasal respiration, eating and speech. Ameloblastic fibro-odontoma consists of elements of ameloblastic odontoma and is more aggressive than the common odontoma.

Radiologically a well-circumscribed lesion presenting as an expansile radiolucency generally contains either a solitary radiopaque mass or multiple small opacities representing the odontoma portion of the lesion (Fig. 5.22). Some of the lesions are relatively small, not over 1 to 2 cm in diameter; while others may be exceedingly large involving a considerable portion of the body of mandible and extending in the ramus.

It is treated by curettage since it does not appear to locally invade bone.

AMELOBLASTIC ODONTOMA

It is also called as 'odonto-ameloblastoma'. It is characterized by the simultaneous occurrence of an ameloblastoma and a composite odontome. It is extremely rare odontogenic tumor.

It causes bony expansion and destruction of the cortex and displacement of teeth and mild pain. It is a slowly expanding lesion of bone which produces considerable facial deformity or asymmetry if left untreated. Mild pain may be present as well as delayed eruption of teeth also occurs.

Radiologically density of Ameloblastic odontoma may be radiopaque and similar to the complex odontoma or may be mixed. There is presence of numerous small radiopaque masses which may or may not bear resemblance to the formed albeit miniature teeth (Fig. 5.23). In some cases, there is only a single irregular radiopaque mass of calcified tissue present. Margin are well defined, uniformly smooth and

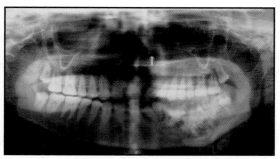

Fig. 5.23: Ameloblastic odontoma presenting as numerous radiopacity inside the radiolucency (*Courtesy:* Dr Amit Parate)

with even border. Central destruction of bone with expansion of the cortical plates is prominent. It can cause bone expansion, destruction and tooth displacement may occur.

Tumor appears to have the same recurrence potential as an ameloblastoma and therefore should be treated similarly.

AMELOBLASTIC FIBROSARCOMA

It is the malignant counterpart of the ameloblastic fibroma in which mesenchymal elements has become malignant. It is also called as 'ameloblastic sarcoma'.

It is uniformly painful, generally grows readily and causes destruction of bone with loosening of teeth. There may be ulceration and bleeding of the overlying mucosa. Swelling is usually soft in consistency.

There is severe bone destruction. It has irregular and poorly defined margins. There may be gross expansion and thinning of cortical bone (Fig. 5.24). In maxillary lesions, the involvement of the antrum may occur.

Radical resection such as hemimandibulectomy or hemimaxillectomy can be done.

MALIGNANT AMELOBLASTOMA

Terminology

Malignant ameloblastoma - are those ameloblastomas that metastasize but in which the metastatic lesion do not show any histological difference from the primary tumor.

Ameloblastic carcinoma - shows obvious histological malignant transformation but the metastatic lesion do not bear resemblance to the primary odontogenic tumor.

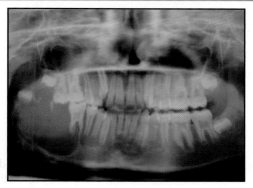

Fig. 5.24: Ameloblastic fibrosarcoma showing
severe bone destruction

Swelling followed by pain and/or rapid growth. Teeth may be displaced and loosened. Tenderness of overlying soft tissue is present. Local extension may occur in adjacent bone, connective tissue or salivary gland.

Radiologically it has well defined border with cortication, presence of crenations or scalloping in the perimeter (Fig. 5.25). There may be loss of cortical boundary and breaching of the cortical boundary with soft tissue spread. It is either unilocular or multilocular giving the appearance of honey comb or soap bubble pattern. Teeth may be displaced and may exhibits root resorption. Lamina dura may be lost. Bony borders may be effaced or breached.

It is treated with en bloc resection. Radiation therapy and chemotherapy for pulmonary metastasis

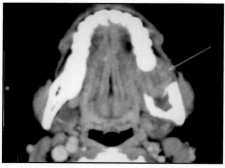

Fig. 5.25: Malignant ameloblastoma (*Courtesy:* Dr N Eswar, Professor and Head, Oral Medicine and Radiology Sri Ramakrishna Dental College and Hospital, Coimbatore, India)

PRIMARY INTRAOSSEOUS CARCINOMA

It is also called as 'central mandibular carcinoma', primary intra-osseous carcinoma', primary epithelial tumor of the jaw, 'primary intra-alveolar epidermoid carcinoma' and central squamous cell carcinoma'. It develops within the depth of the jaw.

The early symptom is swelling of the jaw with pain and mobility of the teeth before ulceration has occurred. Pathological fracture and lip paresthesia also occurs. There is rapid expansion and destruction of jaw bones. Tumor invades the periodontal ligament and the alveolar bone, destroying it. There may be lymphadenopathy. Surface epithelium is normal. Perforation of cortical plate may occur. Extraction of teeth result in non healing socket and sometimes tumor may protrude from the non-healed socket.

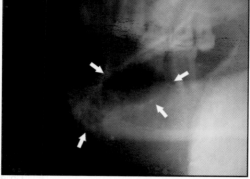

Fig. 5.26: Intraosseous carcinoma presented as diffuse radiolucency in the mandibular molar region (*Courtesy:* Dr Datarkar, Asso. Professor, Oral and Maxillofacial Surgery, SPDC, Wardha India)

Radiologically it presents as a diffuse radiolucency similar to other central malignant neoplasms of the jaws (Fig. 5.26). Mandible is more commonly involve than the maxilla. Molar region is frequently involved than the anterior region. Central squamous cell carcinoma is very rare and appears as more or less rounded radiolucency completely surrounded by bone. Its borders become ragged and there is no evidence of bone formation within the tumor. They are more often rounded or irregular in shape. There is expansion and distortion of the cortical plates of the jaw bone. Teeth that lose both lamina dura and supporting bone appear to be floating in space. There may be perforation of the cortical plate and pathological fracture.

Surgical resection rather than radiotherapy.

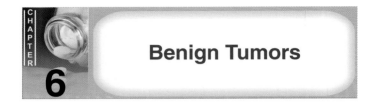

CHAPTER 6

Benign Tumors

Papilloma

It is a relatively common, benign neoplasm of unknown origin, which arises from the surface of epithelium. It may be caused by papilloma virus.

It can be squamous cell papilloma which is congenital, infective, soft papilloma, keratin horns. Other type is called as basal cell papilloma (seborrhoeic or senile wart).

It is a typically an exophytic lesion with a cauliflower-like surface or with finger-like projection. This appearance is caused by presence of deep clefts that extend well into lesion from the surface. It is generally arising from a pedunculated base. Sometime base may be broad rather than pedunculated. There is small mass on mucosa with a papillomatous shape (Fig. 6.1). Tumor in which there is much keratinization is white and lesion without much keratinization are grayish pink in color. Tumor is firm, when keratinized and soft when it is non-keratinized.

It is managed by elliptic incision on the tissue underlying the lesion should be done.

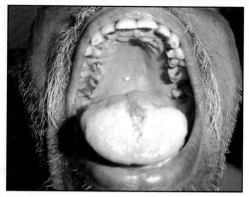

Fig. 6.1: Papilloma seen as papillary small growth in the palate

Pigmented Cellular Nevus

It is also called as 'pigmented mole' or benign melanocytic nevi. Pigmented nevus is a superficial lesion composed of so called nevus cells; hence the term 'cellular nevus'

Nevus is defined as a congenital, developmental tumor like malformation of the skin or mucous membrane.

It can be congenital (small, garment), acquired (intra-dermal nevus, junctional nevus, compound nevus, spindle cell or epitheloid cell nevus and blue (Jadassohn-Tieche) nevus).

Congenital nevi: The congenital nevi, with passage of time, may change from flat, pale tanned macules to elevated, verrucous, hairy lesions.

Intra-dermal nevi: It is more common in children and it is referred as 'common mole'. It may be smooth flat lesion or may be elevated above the surface (Fig. 6.2). It may or may not exhibit brown pigmentation and it often shows strands of hair growing from the surface. It is firm on palpation and rise above the surface.

Junctional nevus: It may appear clinically similar to intra-dermal nevus with distinction chiefly being histological.

Compound nevus: It is firm, raised nodule or polypoid mass. The lesion is composed of two parts intra-dermal and junctional nevus.

Blue nevus: The lesions are smooth and exhibit hair growing from the surface. The color of blue nevi occurs as melanocytes reside deep in the connective tissue and the overlying vessels dampen the brown coloration of melanin and thus yield a blue tint.

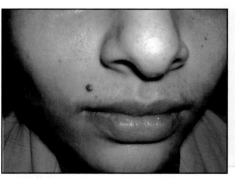

Fig. 6.2: Nevi seen on upper lip as a elevated brown color

Intraorally nevus can occur at any site but most commonly occur on hard palate, buccal mucosa, lips and in gingiva. Most nevi present as raised, macular lesions, but some are flat and macular.

Fibroma

It is a benign soft tissue tumor found in the oral cavity. True benign neoplasm of the fibrous tissue is relatively an infrequent lesion. Most of these lesions are infact hyperplasia or reactive proliferation of fibrous tissue.

They are usually painless, but if they are in a position where they can be bitten or injured, there may be pain and discomfort. It is most often sessile, dome shaped or slightly pedunculated with smooth contour (Figs 6.3 and 6.4). The

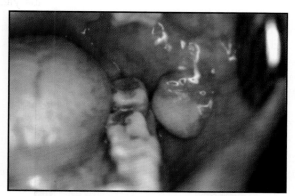

Fig. 6.3: Fibroma presented as dome shaped swelling on the cheek mucosa

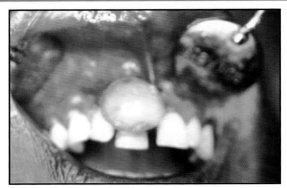

Fig. 6.4: Fibroma presented as sessile growth

lesions on lips and tongue present as circumscribed nodules. Tumor sometimes becomes irritated and inflamed and may show superficial ulceration. The consistency can range from soft and myxomatous to firm and elastic. According to the consistency the tumor is termed as 'hard fibroma' and 'soft fibroma'.

It is treated by conservative excision.

Fibrous Hyperplasia

It is also called as 'inflammatory fibrous hyperplasia', 'denture injury tumor' and 'epulis fissuratum'.

It is caused by ill fitting dentures, ragged margins of teeth, overhanging restorations, sharp spicules of bone, ill fitting clasps and chronic biting of cheek and lips.

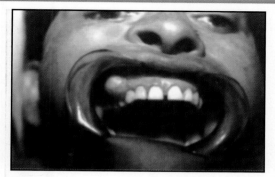

Fig. 6.5: Nodular overgrowth seen in fibrous hyperplasia

There is development of elongated rolls of tissue in the mucolabial or mucobuccal fold area, into which the denture flanges conveniently fit. The proliferation of tissue is usually slow.

There may be small nodular or polypoid overgrowth of fibrous tissue due to gingival irritation (Fig. 6.5).

Epulis fissuratum: When the lesions occur in buccal sulcus due to denture flanges, it is called as epulis fissuratum. In it, there is concomitant overgrowth of surrounding fibrous tissues with a groove in it.

It should be treated with excisional biopsy.

Fibrous Epulis

It is the term used when fibrous growth occurs in the gingiva. The possible cause of it is irritation from subgingival calculus or adjacent carious tooth.

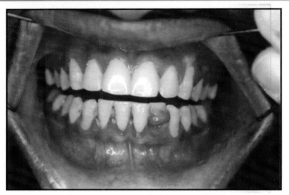

Fig. 6.6: Fibrous epulis seen in relation with lateral incisor which occur due to irritation from calculus

The lesion forms a sessile or pedunculated mass covered by the mucous membrane. It varies from normal tint to deep red, depending upon the vascularity and inflammatory changes (Fig. 6.6). Occasionally superficial ulceration can be seen.

Lesions are excised with small amount of adjacent normal tissue.

Desmoplastic Fibroma

It arises from the mesenchyme of bone. It is also called as 'aggressive fibromatosis'. It produce abundant number of collagen fibers. Swelling of the jaw and sometimes, pain and tenderness may be present (Fig. 6.7). Buccal cortex is

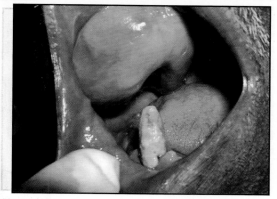

Fig. 6.7: Aggressive fibroma seen in the upper posterior region causing facial asymmetry (*Courtesy:* Dr Amit Parate, Lecturer, Govt. Dental College and Research Center, Nagpur, India)

enlarged and more advanced lesions exhibit facial asymmetry. They are aggressive and proliferate rapidly. It may be associated with Gardner's syndrome.

Radiologically, it appears well defined radiolucency, either unilocular or multilocular. The large lesion appears to be multilocular with very course, thick septa. Smaller lesions are completely radiolucent (Fig. 6.8). It may be poorly or well defined. Divergence of contiguous teeth roots is a common finding. In some cases, there may be root resorption.

Wide local excision is the treatment of choice in these cases.

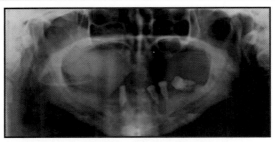

Fig. 6.8: Note the soft tissue radiopacity seen in the upper right region with a radiolucent lesion surrounding it

Chondroma

It is a benign cartilaginous tumor, inspite of the fact that mandible and maxilla are membranous bones, they sometimes contain vestigeal rests of cartilage.

It can be enchondroma or central (develops deep into the bone), ecchondroma (develops on the surface).

It originated from Meckel's cartilage, secondary cartilage like fibrocartilage of mandibular symphysis. It is painless, slowly growing and is locally invasive. Teeth become loose and may be exfoliated. The overlying mucosa is seldom ulcerated.

Radiologically, irregular radiolucent areas whicn can be well defined or ragged or poorly defined. It may develop radiopacities in osteolytic areas, which produce mottled or blurry appearance (Fig. 6.9). Resorption of involved teeth occurs.

It should be excised along with the lining capsule.

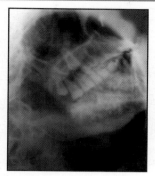

Fig. 6.9: Chondroma appear as mottled appearance

Lipoma

It seldom occurs in oral cavity. It is a benign, slow growing, tumor composed of mature fat cells.

It can be encapsulated lipoma, diffuse lipoma, and lipomatosis.

It appears as a solitary lesion with sessile, pedunculated or submerged base. Size of lesion is approximately 1 cm in diameter. It is well contoured, well defined, round to large ill defined lobulated mass. It grows as round or ovoid mass in oral cavity (Fig. 6.10). It may be lobulated or may be broadly based or have narrow pedicle. Most of the lesions are fluctuant and are not freely movable. Surface is smooth, non tender, soft and cheesy in consistency.

Slip signs—the edge of lipoma is soft, compressible and often slips away from the examining fingers (Fig. 6.11). Transillumination test may be positive.

Surgical excision should be done.

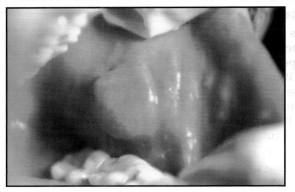

Fig 6.10: Lipoma presented as swelling with smooth surface

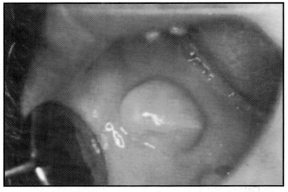

Fig. 6.11: Lipoma presenting with soft edges

Osteoma

It is a benign neoplasm characterized by proliferation of either compact or cancellous bone, usually in an endosteal or periosteal location.

It may arise from cartilage or embryonic periosteum. It arises on the surface of bone as a pedunculated mass. It is located in the medullary bone.

It can be *ivory osteoma* (compact bone), *cancellous osteoma* (trabeculae of bone) and combination.

Ivory osteoma—asymmetry caused by bony hard swelling of jaw (Fig. 6.12). It is usually painless. Mucosa is normal in color and freely movable. Mandibular lesion may

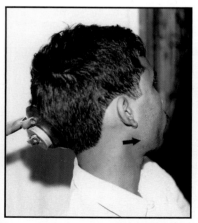

Fig. 6.12: Osteoma of mandible, showing swelling extraorally (*Courtesy:* Dr Datarkar, Asso. Professor, Oral Surgery, SPDC, Wardha, India)

be exophytic extending outwards in soft tissues. Ivory osteoma of the jaw is sometimes pedunculated.

Cancellous osteoma—it is usually pedunculated, although it might have a broad base. The surface may be smooth or slightly irregular.

Radiologically, in ivory osteoma there is small mass of dense bone situated below the level of the root of lower molar. It appears as a uniform radiopaque mass (Fig. 6.13). There may be granular appearance in some cases. It appears as a homogenous density without any internal structure. It has well defined borders. Cancellous type shows evidence of internal trabecular structure. Due to these trabeculations, individual spaces appear to be small.

It is managed by surgical resection.

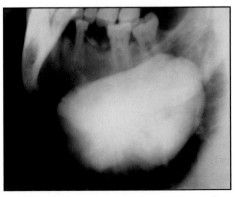

Fig. 6.13: Osteoma presented homogeneous radiopacity

Osteoid Osteoma

It is a variant of osteoblastoma. It is a true neoplasm of osteoblastic derivative. It is small oval or rounded tumor-like nidus which is composed of osteoid and trabeculae of newly formed bone.

The main feature of this neoplasm is severe pain, inspite of the small size of the lesion. Pain usually occurs at night. Soft tissues over the involved bone area may be swollen and tender. It is an oval or round tumor like lesion. There tends to be a marked reaction, which may extend for a considerable distance from the tumor itself.

Radiologically, it appears as small ovoid or round radiolucent area. They are well defined and surrounded by rim of sclerotic bone. The central radiolucency may exhibit some calcification (Fig. 6.14), which manifests in the form of

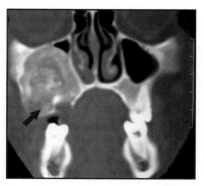

Fig. 6.14: Osteoid osteoma presented with centrally calcification (*Courtesy:* Dr Bhaskar Patle, Lecturer, Oral Medicine and Radiology, SPDC, Wardha, India)

radiopaque foci on radiographs. In occlusal view, the overlying cortex is thickened by new bone being formed subperiosteally.

Severe pain may be relieved by mild obtundants such as aspirin.

Osteochondroma

It is most likely to represent a choristoma, rather than a neoplasm. It is developmental in origin. There is intermingling of two lesions resulting in the term osteochondroma.

It can be central or peripheral types. On the tongue, it appears as a pedunculated swelling of about 1 to 2 cm in the posterior part of the dorsum of tongue, near the foramen cecum. It has broad base. Dysphagia may be the only symptom in this patient. If there is involvement of the condyle, there is difficulty in movements of mandible. Pain is experienced, either in opening and closing the mouth or in deviating the mandible to one side.

Radiologically the radiolucent area in the bone tends to be spherical or oval in shape. Margins of the tumor tend to be more sharply localized and corticated. It shows the presence of bone in the lesion, unlike chondroma which does not show any bone in the lesion. The bone within the tumor is either trabecular or as irregularly shaped amorphous mass (Fig. 6.15).

Peripherally type appears as a protrusion of bone from the surface of the bone. The base of the tumor is usually

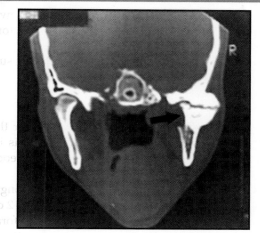

Fig. 6.15: Osteochondroma involving condyle

wide, while the stalk narrows considerably to end in an expansion of variable size.

It consists of surgical removal.

Torus Palatinus

It is also called as 'palatine torus'. It is a slowly growing flat based bony protuberance or excrescence which occurs in the midline of the hard palate. It has been stated that functional stress and genetic factors are important for its origin.

It may be variable in size and shape and be described as flat, spindle shaped, nodular or mushroom like. It is covered

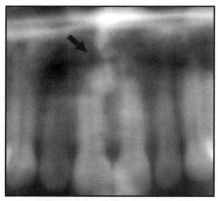

Fig. 6.16: Torus palatinus seen as radiopacity appear over the root of maxillary anterior region

with normal mucosa, which appears pale and occasionally ulcerated, when traumatized.

Radiologically there is relatively dense radiopaque shadow. If the torus has developed in the middle or anterior regions of the palate, it will be superimposed with apical area of maxillary teeth (Fig. 6.16). If it occurs in posterior area, it will appear over the roots of maxillary molars. Borders are well defined as the surface of the torus is of compact bone. Occlusal film that is placed posterior to include the posterior borders of hard palate will provide good demonstration of palatal torus, which will appear oval in shape.

Torus Mandibularis

It is also called as 'mandibular torus'. It is an exostosis or outgrowth of bone found on the lingual surface of the mandible. They consist primarily of compact bone.

There is growth on the lingual surface of the mandible, above the mylohyoid line, usually opposite to the bicuspid teeth (Fig. 6.17). Their size is variable ranging from an outgrowth that is just palpable to one that contacts a torus on the opposite side.

Radiologically radiopaque shadow superimposed over the roots of premolars and molars and occasionally, on the

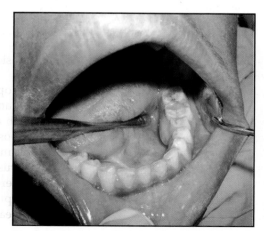

Fig. 6.17: Torus mandibularis seen as an outgrowth on the left lingual of the mandible

incisors and canine. They are sharply demarcated anteriorly, on the periapical film and less dense and less well defined as they extend posteriorly. The shadow tends to be oval with long axis in the posteroanterior direction. On occlusal radiograph, tori appear as radiopaque, homogenous, knobby protuberances from the lingual surface of mandible.

Exostosis

It is also called as 'hyperostoses'. They are small regions of osseous hyperplasia of cortical bone and occasionally, cancellous bone, on the surface of the alveolar process.

Their shape may be nodular, pedunculated or flat protuberance on the surface of bone (Fig. 6.18). They are bony hard on palpation.

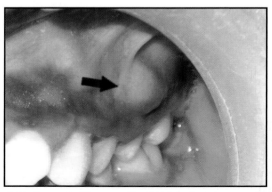

Fig. 6.18: Exostosis (*Courtesy:* Dr Abhishek Soni, Lecturer, Periodontology, VSPM Dental College and Research Center, Nagpur, India)

Radiologically the internal aspect of an exostosis usually is homogenous and radiopaque. They appear as circumscribed, smoothly contoured, rounded radiopaque masses. They are well defined, but some lesions may poorly blend, radiographically into the surrounding bone.

Enostosis

It is also called as '*dense bone island*'. They are internal counterparts of exostosis. They are localized growth of compact bone that extends from the inner surface of cortical bone into the cancellous bone. It is also called as '*whorl*'. A rare condition in which there are thousand of dense islands of bone scattered through the skeleton is known as '*osteopoikile*' or '*osteopoikilosis*' it is asymptomatic.

Radiologically single isolated radiopacities that may be either well defined or diffuse, so that the trabeculae blend with trabacular pattern of adjacent normal bone of jaw. It is more or less rounded, with size varying from a few millimeters upto a centimeter or more (Fig. 6.19).

Hemangioma

It is also called as '*vascular nevus*'. It is a benign tumor which occurs most commonly in vertebrae and skull. It is characterized by proliferation of blood vessels. It is often congenital in origin. It is composed of seemingly disorganized vessels that are filled with blood and is connected to the main vascular system.

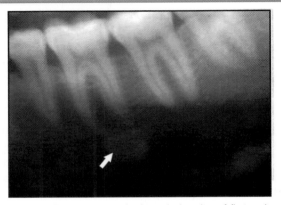

Fig. 6.19: Ensotosis seen in the apical region of first molar

It can be *central* (bone), *capillary hemangioma* (strawberry Angioma, port wine stain, salmon's patch), *cavernous hemangioma* (dilated blood containing spaces, lined by endothelium) and *arterial or plexiform hemangioma* (arteries).

Central - there is non tender expansion of jaws and the swelling is bony hard in consistency (Fig. 6.20). Pain is present in many cases and is probably throbbing in nature. Compressible swelling, which may pulsate and bruit may be detected on auscultation. Anesthesia of skin supplied by mental nerve. Bleeding from gingiva around the neck of affected teeth. Pumping tooth syndrome—it demonstrates pumping action i.e. if the tooth is depressed into the socket, it will rebound into its original position within few minutes. Aspiration of the lesion produces blood. Teeth in affected area may be loosened and may migrate (Fig. 6.21).

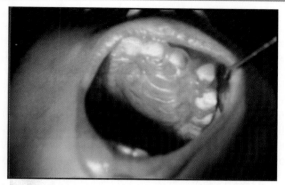

Fig. 6.20: Hemangioma of maxilla central presenting as huge swelling

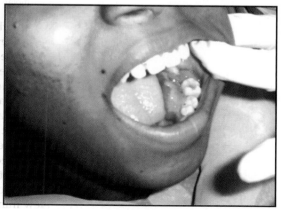

Fig. 6.21: Central hemangioma showing swelling on the gingival tissue (*Courtesy:* Dr Bhaskar Patle, Lecturer Oral Medicine and Radiology SPDC, Wardha, India)

Cavernous appears as a flat or raised lesion of mucosa. It is usually deep red or bluish red and seldom is well circumscribed. Some lesions are pedunculated and globular and some are broad based and flat or slightly raised (Fig. 6.22). Compressibility test is positive. Some times they may increase in size, which can burry the teeth and cause serious deformity and disfigurement.

Port wine stain—red hemangiomas are usually capillary, rather than cavernous variety which is usually more bluish. These reddish macular hemangiomas are called as port wine stain. The port wine stain is generally smooth, but could be slightly raised. It is deep purple-red in color, which may become paler in later life (Fig. 6.23). Color blanches readily on pressure.

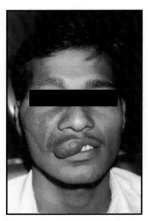

Fig, 6.22: Hemangioma of lip which is red in color

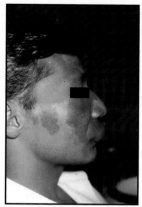

Fig. 6.23: Port wine stain appear as macular lesion

Arterial or plexiform hemangioma—it is a type of congenital arteriovenous fistula. There is a pulsatile swelling of the arteries, veins become tortuous and thick walled; pulsatile feeling like a bag of pulsating earthworms, is elicited.

Radiologically only central hemangioma is visible. It is well defined and corticated and in some cases, it may be ill defined. A moderately well defined zone of radiolucency is present within which the trabecular spaces get enlarged and the trabeculae themselves become coarse and thick. The lesion, therefore, presents typically a multicystic, soap bubble or honeycomb appearance. A structure of the bone is changed in the affected area so that the trabeculae are arranged in a manner which has a rough resemblance to the 'spokes of wheels'.

Roots of teeth are frequently resorbed.

Intralesional injections of sclerosing chemicals, such as 3 percent sodium morrhuate are effective.

LYMPHANGIOMA

It is a benign hamartomatous proliferation of lymphatic vascular tissue. It is a hamartoma, rather than a neoplasm. In it abnormal vessels are filled with clear protein rich fluid containing lymph rather than blood.

It can be superficial or deep.

Usually the disfigurement is notice by the child parents. Occasionally, the vesicles may be rubbed with clothes, get infected and become painful. They are soft masses that dissect along the tissue planes and turn out to be more extensive than anticipated. The surface of the lesion may be smooth or nodular (Figs 6.24 and 6.25). Lesions are subjected to periodic attacks of inflammation which cause the swelling to become larger and tender for the time being. Aspiration yields lymph that is high in lipid. If the tongue is affected, enlargement may occur and the term 'macroglossia' is applied. On the tongue, it is characterized by irregular nodularity of the surface of the tongue with gray and pink, grapelike projection. They are often elevated and nodular in appearance and may have the same color as the surrounding mucosa.

Surgical removal of the bulk of the lesion can be done.

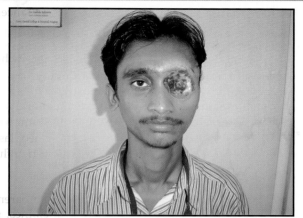

Fig. 6.24: Lymphangioma of left eye. Note the complete obliteration of the left eye caused by the tumor (*Courtesy:* Dr Bhaskar Patle, Lecturer SPDC, Wardha, India)

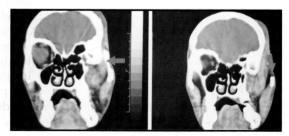

Fig. 6.25: Lymphangioma of the left eye causing complete obliteration of the eye (*Courtesy:* Dr Bhaskar Patle, lecturer Oral Medicine and Radiology, SPDC, Wardha, India)

ARTERIOVENOUS FISTULA

It also called as 'arteriovenous shunt' or 'arteriovenous malformation'. It is a direct communication between an artery and vein that bypasses the intervening capillary bed. It may be congenital or acquired. A lesion with a thrill or bruit, or with an obviously warmer surface, is most likely a special vascular malformation, called arteriovenous malformation, with direct flow of blood from the venous to the arterial system, bypassing the capillary beds.

It can be *cirsoid aneurysm, varicose aneurysm, Ane`1urysm varix.*

There is mass of extraosseous soft tissue swelling. It is having purplish discoloration. Bone may be expanded. Pulse may be detected on auscultation and aspiration produces blood.

Radiologically it causes a resorptive radiolucent lesion. They are well defined and corticated. It is multilocular (Fig. 6.26). Walls of shunt may contain apparent calcified material.

It should be treated by surgical excision.

Neurofibroma

It is also called as 'neurofibromatosis, 'Von Reckling-hausen's disease of skin' or 'fibroma Molluscum'. It is inherited as a simple autosomal dominant trait with variable penetrance.

It may appear as numerous sessile or pedunculated, elevated smooth surfaced nodules of variable size, which are scattered over the skin surface. In other forms, there are

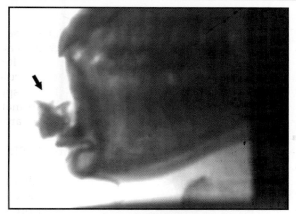

Fig. 6.26: Arteriovenous fistula presented as radiolucency with corticated margin and some degree of calcification

deeper, more diffuse lesions which are often of greater proportion than superficial nodules and are sometimes referred to as 'elephantiasis neuromatosa'. In some cases, loose overgrowth of thickened, pigmented skin may hang in folds (Fig. 6.27). In addition majority of the patients exhibit asymmetric areas of cutaneous pigmentation, often described as "cafe-au-lait" spots.

Orally the central lesion may have multiple lesions, occurring in both jaws simultaneously, expanding and filling the maxillary sinus. There are discrete, non-ulcerated nodules, which tend to be of the same color as the normal mucosa. It may produce pain or paraesthesia, if associated with mandibular nerve.

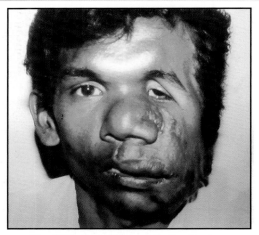

Fig. 6.27: Neurofibroma affecting the face
as pedunculated mass

Radiologically there is an area of bone destruction which presents a radiolucent shadow of varying density, depending on the amount of bone that has been replaced by tumor (Fig. 6.28). Margins of radiolucency are well defined, curved and may be hyperostotic. In neurofibroma of inferior dental nerve shows fusiform or more or less circular enlargement of mandibular canal. In some cases there may be an elongated lesion with an undulating border.

Solitary lesion may be surgically excised.

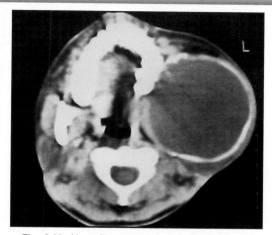

Fig. 6.28: Neurofibroma presented as radiolucent
lesion surrounded by hyperostotic border

Neurilemmoma

It is also called as 'schwannoma', 'perineural fibroblastoma',
'neurinoma' and 'lemmoma'. It is of neuroectodermal origin,
arising from Schwann cells that make the inner layer
covering the peripheral nerves.

Usual complain is lump in jaw, in case of central tumor
and single circumscribed nodule, in case of soft tissue
lesions. Paraesthesia may be associated, which occurs
anterior to the tumor. Pain is localized to the tumor site. The
mass is firm on palpation. It is non-productive to aspiration.

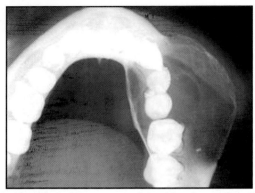

Fig. 6.29: Neurilemmoma seen on right side of mandible (*Courtesy:* Dr Karthikeya Patil, Professor and Head, Oral Medicine and Radiology, JSS Dental College and Hospital, Mysore, India)

The radiolucent area is usually located within the expanded inferior alveolar nerve, posterior to the mental foramen. Round to oval radiolucent area of bone destruction (Fig. 6.29). There may be crescent shaped cystic radiolucency. Margins of the lesions are well defined and hyperostotic. It may cause root resorption of adjacent teeth. If the tumor protrudes from the mental foramina, erosive lesion of the surface of jaw bone occurs.

Surgical excision is the treatment of choice.

Neuroma

It is also called as 'amputation neuroma' or 'traumatic neuroma'. It is not a true neoplasm, but an exuberant attempt at repair of a damaged nerve trunk.

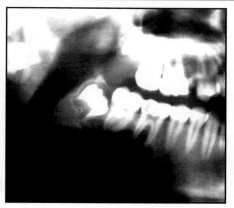

Fig. 6.30: Neuroma with well defined and corticated borders

It appears as a small nodule or swelling of the mucosa. Due to the pressure applied by enlargement of the tangled mass in its bony cavity, severe pain may be experience.

Radiologically it is seen as a destructive lesion. It appears as a radiolucent area (Fig. 6.30). It has got well defined and corticated borders. Some expansion of the canal is seen.

Simple excision of nodule along with proximal portion of the involved nerve.

Peripheral Giant Cell Granuloma

It is also called as 'peripheral giant cell reparative granuloma', 'giant cell epulis', 'osteoclastoma' and 'peripheral giant cell tumor'.

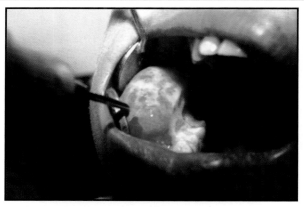

Fig. 6.31: Peripheral giant cell granuloma presenting as hour glass appearance in oral cavity

It can occur due injury, chronic infection and hormonal. Early lesion appears as discoloration and slight swelling of the buccal aspect of the gingiva. Later the lesion increase in size and becomes rounded and very often pedunculated. Sometimes, it grows in an hour-glass manner (Fig. 6.31), with the waist of the lesion between two teeth and the globular extremities presenting buccally and lingually. The color of the lesion is usually dark red or maroon color. Lesions with much fibrous tissue are paler (Fig. 6.32). It may feel soft to hard. It is vascular or hemorrhagic and sometimes ulceration is also present. There may be tenderness on palpation.

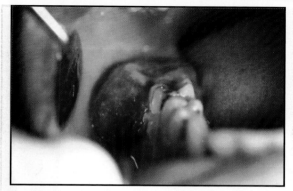

Fig. 6.32: Vascular type of peripheral giant cell granuloma presenting with ulceration

Radiologically in edentulous areas, the peripheral giant cell granuloma characteristically exhibits superficial erosion of the bone with peripheral 'cuffing' of the bone.

Excision with borders of normal tissue with entire base of the lesion, so that recurrence is avoided.

Pyogenic Granuloma

It is also called as 'granuloma pyogenicum'. It is a response of tissues to non-specific infection of staphylococcus or streptococci. It is relatively a common soft tissue tumor of the skin and mucus membrane. It is known to be a reactive inflammatory process in which there is an exuberant fibro vascular proliferation of the connective tissue, secondary to some low grade chronic irritant.

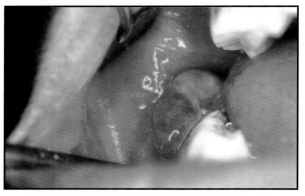

Fig. 6.33: Pyogenic granuloma presenting as sessile growth with exudation of purulent material

It is an asymptomatic papular, nodular polypoid mass. Lesions are elevated, pedunculated or sessile masses with smooth (Fig. 6.33), lobulated or even warty surface, which commonly ulcerates and shows tendency to hemorrhage upon slightest pressure or trauma. It has red and white pattern. It is deep red to reddish purple depending on the vascularity; painless and rather soft in consistency, with some lesions having brown cast, if hemorrhage has occurred into the tissues.

Surgical excision and care is taken to remove the calculus of adjacent teeth as it may act as a local irritant and cause recurrence.

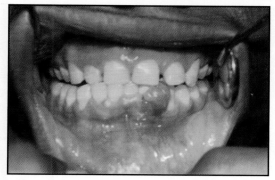

Fig. 6.34: Pregnancy tumor presented as well defined lesion

Pregnancy Tumor

It occurs as a result of local minor trauma and in cases where tissue reaction is intensified by endocrine alteration occurring during pregnancy.

It is a well defined lesion, which gradually increases in size and may or may not regress after delivery (Fig. 6.34). If surgically removed during pregnancy, it usually recurs.

Radiologically, in some of the cases there is slight rarefaction of the bone beneath the attachment of the tumor, usually at the crest of the alveolus.

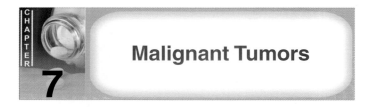

CHAPTER 7

Malignant Tumors

PERIPHERAL SQUAMOUS CELL CARCINOMA

It is also called as 'epidermoid carcinoma' or 'epithelioma'. The majority of oral cancer cases are of squamous cell carcinoma. The oral lesion often invades the jaw. It arises in gingival tissue, buccal sulcus, floor of mouth and some other portion of oral mucosa.

Patient may present with awareness of a mass in the mouth and neck. Small lesion is asymptomatic. Large lesions may cause pain or paresthesia and swelling. Patients complain of persistent ulcer in the oral cavity. Function of organ is impaired. The clinical appearance of a carcinomatous ulcer is that one of irregular shape, induration and raised everted edges (Fig. 7.1).

Usually have broad base and are dome like or nodular. Surface may range from granular to pebbly to deeply creviced. In some cases, surface may be entirely necrotic and have ragged whitish gray appearance (Fig. 7.2). It may be completely red or red surface may be sprinkled with white necrotic or keratin area (Figs 7.3 and 7.4). Base and borders

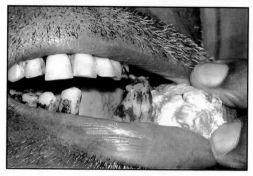

Fig. 7.1: Malignancy having whitish pebbled appearance seen on buccal mucosa (*Courtesy:* Dr Suhas Darvekar, Mumbai)

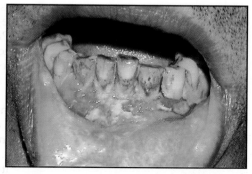

Fig. 7.2: Irregular shaped ulcer seen in gingiva due to malignancy

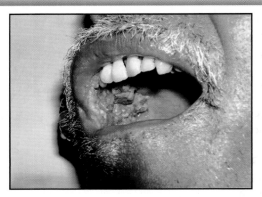

Fig. 7.3: Ulcerated growth seen on buccal mucosa

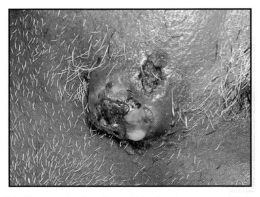

Fig. 7.4: Same patient in figure 7.3 showing extraoral extension

are firm to palpate and the lesion may get fixed after infiltration into underlying tissues.

Lymph nodes: Superficial and deep cervical nodes are commonly affected. They become enlarged and are firm to hard on palpation. The nodes are non-tender unless associated with secondary infection or an inflammatory response. It may be nodular or polypoid. Fixation of nodes to adjacent tissues occurs later.

Carcinoma of Floor of Mouth

The typical carcinoma of the floor of mouth is an indurated ulcer of varying size, on one side of the midline. It may take form of wart like growth (Fig. 7.5), which tend to spread superficially rather than in depth. The proximity of this tumor to the tongue produces some limitation of motion of

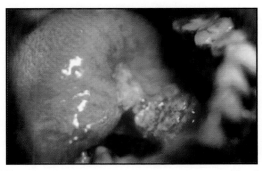

Fig. 7.5: Carcinoma of floor of mouth showing on one side of midline

these organs, often induces peculiar slurring of the speech. There may be excessive salivation. Metastasis from the floor of the mouth is found most commonly in the sub-maxillary group of lymph nodes.

Carcinoma of Buccal Mucosa

The tumor begins as small nodules and enlarges to form a wart like growth which ultimately ulcerates (Fig. 7.6). Extension into the muscle of neck, alveolar mucosa and ultimately into bone may occur. The most common site of metastasis is the submaxillary lymph nodes.

Carcinoma of Palate

Palatal cancer usually manifest as a poorly defined ulcerated painful lesion on one side of the midline. Most of

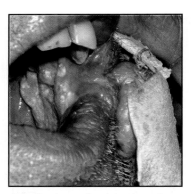

Fig. 7.6: Carcinoma involving buccal mucosa
(*Courtesy:* Dr Suhas Darvekar, Mumbai)

the lesions are exophytic and with broad base and nodular surface (Figs 7.7 and 7.8). It frequently crosses the midline and may extend laterally to include tonsillar pillars or even the uvula. The tumor of hard palate may invade the bone or occasionally the nasal cavity while infiltrating lesions of the soft palate may extend into the nasopharynx.

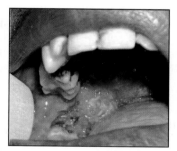

Fig. 7.7: Squamous cell carcinoma affecting palate showing ulceration
(*Courtesy:* Dr Suhas Darvekar, Mumbai)

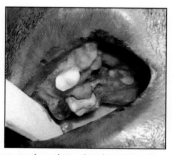

Fig 7.8: Malignancy in palate showing extensive ulceration and displacement of teeth

Radiographic Features

There is roughly semicircular or saucer shaped erosion into the bone surface. There is presence of ragged ill define borders that illustrate the varying uneven osteolytic invasion. Rarely the border may appear smooth without the cortex indicating underlining erosion rather than invasion. If pathological fracture occurs, the borders show sharpened thinned bone ends with displacement of segments and adjacent soft tissue mass (Fig. 7.9).

Little 'bays' of bone destruction extend into the bone, leaving irregular promontories of variable length and width extending into the main area of bone destruction. Margins of 'bays' are irregular and jagged (Fig. 7.10). These produce a finger like projection and this appearance is described as infiltration of the bone.

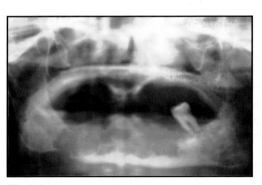

Fig. 7.9: Excessive destruction of bone also showing pathological fracture on right side

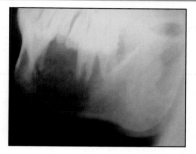

Fig. 7.10: Malignancy showing irregular destruction with ill
defined margin in the periphery

The inferior border of mandible may be thinned or destroyed. Teeth appear to float in a mass of radiolucent soft tissue bereft of any bony support. In extensive tumor soft tissue mass may grow into the teeth and teeth appear to be grossly displaced from its normal position.

It is managed by radical surgery, radiation and chemotherapy.

Metastatic Carcinoma

It is also called as 'secondary carcinoma'. It is the most common malignant tumor in the skeleton. This tumor is transported to an area distant from its origin and establishes a new foot holds and are said to have metastasized. Although the metastatic carcinoma of jaw is uncommon, its recognition is important because the jaw tumors may be the first indication that the patient has a malignant disease.

Oral diagnostician can make an invaluable contribution of pathologic process of bone. Most common sites of origin are breast, lung, kidney, thyroid, prostate and colon.

Mandible is involved much more frequently than maxilla, especially in the region near premolars and molars as tumor metastasizes to those bones which are rich in hemopoietic marrow. Early lesion is nodule or dome with shaped smooth surface and due to trauma may get ulcerated (Fig. 7.11). There may be pain followed by paresthesia or anesthesia of lip or chin. Teeth in this region may become loose or exfoliate and root resorption may occur. On occasion, tumor may breach the outer cortical plate of jaws and extend into surrounding soft tissue or presents as an intraoral mass.

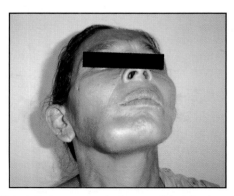

Fig. 7.11: Metastatic tumor seen in the mandible (*Courtesy:* Dr Bhaskar Patle, Lecturer, Oral Medicine and Radiology, SPDC, Wardha, India)

Radiologically it can be osteolytic (Fig. 7.12) (ill defined radiolucent destructive lesion may be single or multiple and vary in size) or osteoblastic (Fig. 7.13) (Irregular 'salt and pepper appearance' can be seen in some cases).

It is managed by chemotherapy, radiation therapy, surgery, immunotherapy and hormone therapy.

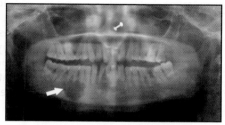

Fig. 7.12: Metastatic carcinoma presented as a unilocular radiolucency in the mandible on right side (*Courtesy:* Dr Bhaskar Patle, Lecturer, Oral Medicine and Radiology, SPDC, Wardha, India)

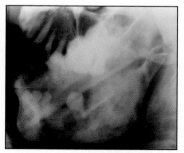

Fig. 7.13: Osteoblastic variety of metastatic tumor (*Courtesy:* Dr Ashok L, Professor and Head, Oral Medicine and Radiology, Bapuji, Dental College and Hospital, Davanagere, India)

Basal Cell Carcinoma

It is also called as *'basal cell epithelioma'* or *'Rodent ulcer'*. It arises from basal layer of epidermis or from the hair follicle.

It is caused by *prolonged exposure to sunlight*, burn scars and ionizing radiation.

It begins as a small, slightly elevated papule which ulcerates, heals over and then breaks down again to form crusted ulcer. It develops a smooth, rolled border representing tumor cells spreading laterally beneath the skin (Fig. 7.14). Untreated lesion continues to enlarge and infiltrate the adjacent and deeper tissues and it may even erode deeply into the cartilage or bone. Due to it's invading and destructive

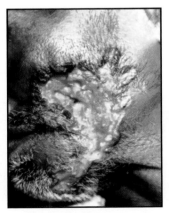

Fig. 7.14: Basal cell carcinoma showing rodent ulcer type lesion showing invasion

infiltration into adjoining tissues, it gradually increases in size and accounts for its synonym 'rodent ulcer'. It is never seen in oral cavity unless it arrives there by invasion and infiltration from a skin surface. Occasionally, it may metastasize to lymph nodes.

Surgical excision or x-ray radiation can be given.

Malignant Melanoma

It is a neoplasm of epidermal melanocytes. It is one of the biologically unpredictable and deadly of all human neoplasms. Sunlight is very important etiological factor in cutaneous melanoma.

It can be superficial spreading melanoma, nodular melanoma and lentigo maligna melanoma.

Superficial spreading melanoma—it begins as pigmented macule, restricted mostly to epithelium and junction. In advanced cases, melanoma present as an ulcerated (Fig. 7.15), fungating growth which is associated with bleeding.

Nodular melanoma—It is firm on palpation. It has got erythematous borders which surround the tumor. There is rapid infiltration in nodular type of melanoma. It may be focal or diffuse. Many times it may ulcerate and hemorrhage may be seen.

Lentigo maligna melanoma—it is pigment macule with ill defined margins. It occurs characteristically as a macular lesion of the skin.

Orally the lesions usually appear as deeply pigmented areas, at times ulcerated and hemorrhagic (Fig. 7.16), which

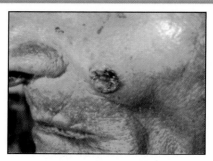

Fig. 7.15: Superficial spreading melanoma seen as ulcerated growth

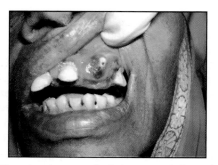

Fig. 7.16: Malignant melanoma affecting upper anterior region (*Courtesy:* Dr Amit Parate, Lecturer, Oral Medicine and Radiology, Government Dental College and Hospital, Nagpur)

tend to increase progressively in size. The lesion presents as a soft, darkish brown or black mass. It may have a nodular or a papillary surface. The tumor causes extensive destruction of the underlying bone.

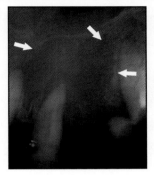

Fig. 7.17: Malignant melanoma affecting upper anterior region see the irregular bone loss (*Courtesy:* Dr Amit Parate, Lecturer, Government Dental College and Hospital, Nagpur)

Radiologically it has got ill defined margin (Fig. 7.17).

There may be ulcerations and bleeding of the oral mucosa. It is treated by surgical irradiation, immunotherapy and by chemotherapy or, by combination of these methods.

Verrucous Carcinoma

It is a slow growing low-grade carcinoma. Tobacco chewers have high percentage of these cases. It occurs usually in a person habitual to hold the quid in the buccal sulcus.

They appear papillary in nature with pebbly surface (Fig. 7.18) which is sometimes covered by a white leukoplakic film. They have rugae-like folds with deep cleft between them. In some cases, there may be warty fungating mass. Margins are well defined and show rim of slightly

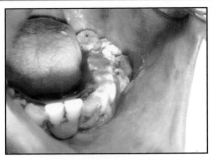

Fig. 7.18: Verrucous carcinoma involving the buccal sulcus. Note the papillary nature of the lesion (*Courtesy:* Dr Bhaskar Patle, Lecturer SPDC Wardha, Nagpur, India)

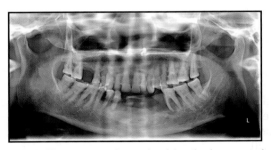

Fig. 7.19: Verrucous carcinoma involving the lower anterior region causing erosion of the bone in that area

elevated normal mucosa. Pain and difficulty in mastication are common complain. Regional lymph nodes are often tender and enlarged simulating metastatic tumor, but the node involvement is usually inflammatory.

Radiologically there is erosion of bone in affected region (Fig. 7.19).

Wide surgical excision—excision must be sufficiency radical to remove the entire lesion.

FIBROSARCOMA

It is malignant neoplasm composed of malignant fibroblast that produces collagen and elastin.

It produces fleshy bulky mass of tissue. There may be pain and loosening of the teeth. Sensory neural abnormalities may occur if it involves peripheral nerves. Initially they resemble benign fibrous outgrowth, but they grow rapidly to produce large tumor. Large tumors are prone to ulceration and hemorrhage. Secondary infections are seen in some cases. In some cases, pathological fracture may occur.

Destructive lesion may stimulate the osteolytic form of osteosarcoma. They are poorly demarcated, noncorticated and lack any resemblance of capsule. They tend to elongate through marrow space. If soft tissue lesions occur adjacent to bone, they cause a saucer like depression in the underlying bone or invade it: as in the case of squamous cell carcinoma (Fig. 7.20). Teeth are displaced and loose their supporting bone so that they appear to be floating in space. Lamina dura and follicular cortices are obliterated. In some cases, periodontal space widening may occur.

Radical surgical excision is most commonly used treatment modality.

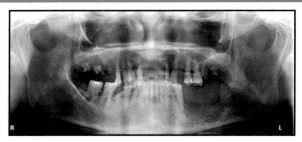

Fig. 7.20: Fibrosarcoma showing saucer like destruction of the bone

CHONDROSARCOMA

It is also called as '*chondrogenic sarcoma*'. It develops from natural cartilage or a benign cartilaginous tumor.

It can be *primary* (arise from the cartilage) and *secondary* (benign cartilaginous tumor).

It is painless in early stages with facial asymmetry as first complain but as it enlarges swelling becomes bony hard and painful (Fig. 7.21). There may be headache. Teeth adjacent to the lesion are resorbed, loosened and get exfoliated. In some cases, there may be hemorrhage from the neck of teeth. There may be sensory nerve deficit, proptosis and visual disturbances. Mucosal covering appears normal in early stage but later it ulcerates and develops necrotic surface, if chronically traumatized. If it occurs in/or near the temporomandibular joint region, trismus and abnormal joint function may result.

Radiologically it may be sclerotic or mixed, if there is calcification of neoplastic tissue. Lytic lesions with poorly defined borders (Fig. 7.22). The lesion is rounding, ovoid or

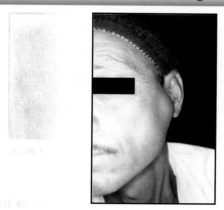

Fig. 7.21: Chondrosarcoma of condyle showing
swelling in the condylar region

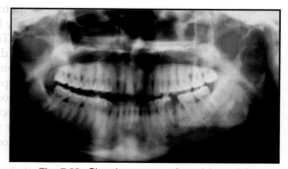

Fig. 7.22: Chondrosarcoma of condyle on left
side of condyle showing complete destruction

lobulated. It may be multiloculated or develop as multiple radiolucency containing radiopaque foci. The center radiopaque structure has been described as 'flocculent', implying snowlike features. In some cases we may get soap bubble appearance, ground glass or granular appearance, sun ray appearance, speckled appearance.

There may be band like widening of periodontal ligament space; resorption of root may occur. lesion on the condyle cause it's expansion and remodeling of the corresponding articular fossa and eminence. If the lesion occurs in the articular disc region, a widened joint space may be present with corresponding remodeling of condylar neck.

Surgery is the only treatment of choice and there is 5 years survival rat.

Osteosarcoma

It is also called as 'osteogenic sarcoma'. It is the most common malignant tumor of bone. It is derived from osteoblasts in which tumor cells contain high level of alkaline phosphatase.

It can cause by radiation therapy, traumatic irritation, fibro-osseous diseases, genetic mutation and some viral causes.

It grows rapidly with a doubling time of 32 days and shows recurrence and early metastasis via blood stream to lungs. There is exophthalmos, blindness, nasal obstruction and epistaxis.

Orally swelling of a short history and is accompanied by pain. Affected tooth may become displaced or loose. Numbness of lip and chin due to involvement of inferior alveolar nerve. There may be trismus and hemorrhage. Expansion is very firm due to dense fibrous tissue (Figs 7.23 and 7.24). Later, the surface gets ulcerated and looks like whitish grey in color.

Radiologically there is symmetrical widening of periodontal ligament space in early stage of the disease. It may develop into a frankly osteolytic stage, mixed stage, i.e. those which produce some bone and osteoblastic stage which are almost entirely bone forming.

Osteolytic stage—lesions are unicentric and borders of the lesion are ill defined. There is moth eaten appearance.

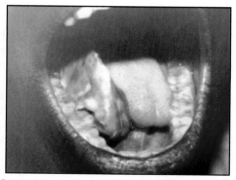

Fig. 7.23: Osteosarcoma of mandible presented as mass inside the oral cavity (*Courtesy:* Dr Datarkar. Asso. Professor, Oral and Maxillofacial Surgery, SPDC, Wardha, India)

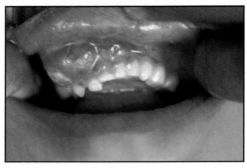

Fig. 7.24: Osteosarcoma seen inside the oral cavity as an expansile growth (*Courtesy:* Dr Lambade, Asso. Professor, Oral and Maxillofacial Surgery, CDC, Ragnandgao, India)

Perforation and expansion of cortical margins occurs. Adjacent lamina dura may be destroyed.

Mixed—the presence of new bone laid down deep to the periosteum may be slight or it may be gross. There is evidence of bone formation as well as destruction. In some cases there is a well defined area of bone destruction, with partially corticated borders and some bone within the tumor itself (Fig. 7.25). Honey comb appearance—the bone within the radiolucent area of destruction may take the form of strands, which may be few and intersecting, or may produce a more or less honeycomb appearance.

Osteoblastic: *Granular appearance, Sun ray appearance Codman's* triangle (Fig. 7.26) (two triangular radiopacities project from the cortex and mark the lateral extremities of the lesion referred as 'Codman's triangle').

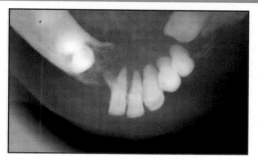

Fig. 7.25: Osteogenic sarcoma of mixed variety

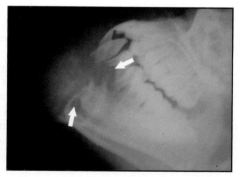

Fig. 7.26: Osteogenic sarcoma showing sunray appearance

Radical resection with amputation of bone can be carried out and sometimes adjuvant chemotherapy can be instituted.

Ewing's Sarcoma

It was first described in 1921 by James Ewing. It is also called as 'round cell sarcoma' or 'endothelial myeloma'. It is derived from mesenchymal connective tissue of bone marrow.

Initially, intermittent pain occurs which later becomes continuous and is associated with rapid growth of the tumor and enlargement of bone. It is associated with febrile attacks and leukocytosis. The swelling is hard but occasionally it may be soft and fluctuant. When the tumor breaks through the cortex, it spreads extensively in the soft tissues and form a soft mass which may ulcerate. The patient may have low grade fever, facial neuralgias, lip paresthesia. Teeth may become mobile and paresthesia may develop.

Radiologically it is ill defined destructive radiolucent, lesion which may be unilocular or multilocular (Fig. 7.27).

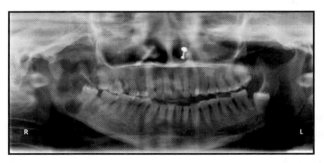

Fig. 7.27: Ewing's sarcoma seen as a multilocular radiolucency with ill-defined border and associated pathological fracture

It has ill defined margins and is never corticated. In advanced cases, bone is destroyed in uneven fashion, resulting in ragged borders. Areas of sclerosis may be found around the margins of the lesion with mottled rarefaction. Onion skin appearance, Sun ray appearance can occur. It may cause pathologic fracture. There may be destruction of lamina dura and the supporting bone of adjacent teeth.

Surgery, X-ray radiation can be used but survival period is very less.

HODGKIN'S LYMPHOMA

It was first described by British pathologist Thomas Hodgkin in 1832. It is characterized by painless enlargement of lymphoid tissue throughout the body.

The involved nodes are painless. Generalized weakness, loss of weight, cough, dyspnea and anorexia are seen. Pain in back and abdomen owing to splenic enlargement, due to pressure of enlarged nodes or involvement of vertebrae. The lymph nodes are discrete and rubbery in consistency with overlying skin being freely mobile. Splenomegaly is usually seen in later stage. Characteristic features of this disease are *Pel-Ebstein fever*, a cyclic spiking of high fever and generalized severe pruritis of unknown etiology.

Orally it may appear in the oral cavity as an ulcer or a swelling or as an intra-bony lesion which presents as a hard swelling.

Radiologically malignant lymphoma arising in the oral cavity does spreads to bone and cause irregular bone loss to the area of the lesion.

It is managed by *radiotherapy, chemotherapy, Splenectomy.*

Non-Hodgkin's Lymphoma

It is also called as 'lymphosarcoma'. In this group, there is neoplastic proliferation of lymphoid cells, usually affecting the B-lymphocytes. Unlike Hodgkin's lymphoma, the disease is frequently widespread at the time of diagnosis, often involving not only the lymph nodes but also bone marrow, spleen and other tissue. Early involvement of bone marrow is typical of this lymphoma.

It can be nodular or diffuse. It is caused by Viral (herpes) or immunological.

The patient complains of tiredness, loss of weight, fever and sweating. Pain is the main symptom of bone involvement which may present as a pathological fracture. Patient may complain abdominal pain, nausea, vomiting, diarrhea or intestinal obstruction which may occur due to involvement of gastrointestinal tract.

Orally palatal lesions have been described as slow growing, painless, bluish soft tissues mass which may be confused with minor salivary gland tumors. Paresthesia of mental nerve has been reported.

Radiologically small radiolucent foci scattered throughout the area may be seen. Subsequent radiographs of the expanding lesion will show that these small foci have coalesced to form large multilocular moth eaten radiolucency with poorly defined margins.

Chemotherapy, radiotherapy and transplantation of autologous stem cell.

Leukemia

It is also called as 'leucosis'. It is defined as a neoplastic proliferation of WBC in bone marrow, usually in circulating blood and sometimes in other organs such as liver, spleen and lymph nodes. Presence of leukemic cells in bone marrow results in impairment of normal hemopoiesis with resultant anemia, granulocytopenia and thrombocytopenia.

It can be acute lymphoblastic leukemia, acute non lymphoblastic or myeloid leukemia, chronic lymphatic leukemia, and chronic myeloid leukemia.

It is caused by virus (Epstein Barr virus, herpes) radiation and atomic energy, chemical agents (aniline dyes; benzene and phenylbutazone), anticancer drugs (melphalan and chlorambucil), genetic and chromosomal factors and Immunological deficiency syndrome.

Acute leukemia—symptoms usually result from bone marrow suppression and infiltration of other organs and tissues by leukemic cells. Weakness, fever, headache, generalized swelling of lymph nodes, petechiae or hemorrhage in skin and mucus membrane are seen. Bone pain and tenderness, resulting from marrow expansion, with infiltration of subperiosteum. The clinical features are due to anemia and thrombocytopenia viz pallor, dyspnea, fatigue, petechiae, ecchymosis, epistaxis and melena. Orally Paresthesia of lower lip and chin may be present. There may be toothache due to leukemic cell infiltration of dental pulp. The oral mucous membrane shows pallor, ulceration with necrosis (Fig. 7.30), petechiae, ecchymosis and bleeding tendency (Figs 7.28 and 7.29). There may be massive necrosis

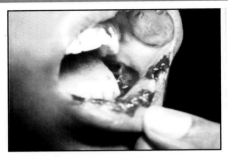

Fig. 7.28: Bleeding from lip occur in patient with leukemia

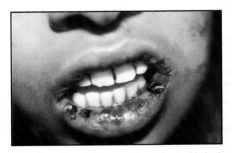

Fig. 7.29: Crusting of lip occur in patient with leukemia

of lingual mucosa with sloughing. Gingiva shows hypertrophy and cyanotic discoloration. It is managed by chemotherapeutic agents.

Chronic leukemias—these are characterized by the presence of large leukemic cells and differentiated WBCs in the bone marrow, peripheral blood and other tissues. It has

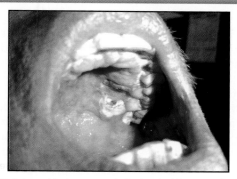

Fig. 7.30: Intraoral lesions seen in leukemia (*Courtesy:* Dr Bhaskar Patle, Lecturer, Oral Medicine and Radiology, SPDC, Wardha, India)

a prolonged clinical course even without therapy. There may be slowly advancing anemia with loss of weight, prominence of abdomen and discomfort in the left upper quadrant due to splenomegaly. Anemia causes weakness, fatigue and dyspnea on exertion. As the disease progress thrombocytopenia can cause petechiae, ecchymosis as well as hemorrhage from the skin and mucus membrane. Liver may be enlarged but lymph nodes are normal. It is managed by chemotherapy.

Radiologically it is presented as ill defined patchy radiolucent area. This patchy area may coalesce to from larger areas of ill defined radiolucent regions. Moth eaten appearance, sclerosis of bone, onion peel appearance. There is also loss of lamina dura with loosening of teeth.

MULTIPLE MYELOMA

It is also called as 'myelomatosis'. It is a malignant neoplasm of plasma cells of the bone marrow with widespread involvement of the skeletal system, including the skull and jaws.

It is thought to be multicentric in origin. There is proliferation of a single clone of abnormal plasma cells in the bone marrow. Skeletal pain associated with motion or pressure over the tumor masses, is an early symptom. Spontaneous pathological fracture with acute pain may be present. Weakness and pain of back and thorax also may be presenting symptoms. Pain in the involved bone may be aggregated by exercise and relieved by rest. The patient may also complain of tiredness, bleeding tendency and bruising of skin due to anemia and thrombocytopenia. The cause of bleeding is that the abnormal globulins bind with coagulation factors which also increase the viscosity of blood. Patient may complain of vomiting due to increase serum calcium level.

There is an increased susceptibility to infection due to abnormal immunoglobulin production by the plasma cells.

Orally the patient may experience pain, swelling and numbness of the jaw. Epulis formation or unexplained mobility of teeth is also detectable. Intraoral swelling tends to be ulcerated, rounded and bluish red similar to a peripheral giant cell lesion. Sometimes, swelling may erode buccal plate and produce rubbery expansion of jaw. Chronic trauma produces an inflamed and ulcerative necrotic surface. Secondary signs of bone marrow involvement such

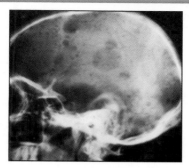

Fig. 7.31: Multiple myeloma presented as punched out radiolucency seen in skull (*Courtesy:* Dr A K Ganju, Clinical Hematologist, Nagpur, India)

as pallor of oral tissue, intraoral hemorrhage and susceptibility to infection may also be seen.

Radiologically in the radiograph, it appears as a small rounded and discrete radiolucency having punched out appearance (Fig. 7.31). There may be numerous areas of bone destruction within the region of generalized radiolucency. Diffuse destructive lesions of bone may occur. It has well defined margins and lack the circumferential osteosclerotic activity. In some cases, borders of the lesion may display a thin sclerotic rim and even areas of opacification. Lamina dura and follicle of impacted teeth may loose their typical corticated surrounding bone in a manner analogous to that seen in hyperparathyroidism.

It is managed by *chemotherapeutic agents, blood transfusion, cell transplantation radiotherapy, Biphosphonate therapy.*

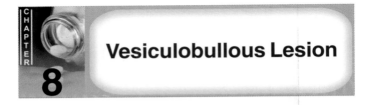

C
H
A
P
T
E
R

8

Vesiculobullous Lesion

TRAUMATIC ULCER

It is a frequently encountered ulcerative lesion of mouth. The common term used to denote a traumatic ulcer is *'decubitus ulcer', 'tropic ulcer', 'neutronstropic'* and *'Bednar's ulcer'*.

It is caused by mechanical or physical (biting, sharp or mal-posed teeth or roots, sharp food, stiff tooth brush bristles, sharp margins of crown, fillings, denture, orthodontic appliances and faulty instrumentation), chemical (caustic substances such as silver nitrate, phenol, TCA, formocresol, eugenol, eucalyptus oil, phosphorus and acetylsalicylic acid), thermal (excessive heat in the form of hot fluid or food, on rare occasion the application of the dry ice, reverse smoking and hot instrumentation) and *electrical current*.

The appearance of the traumatic ulcer varies markedly depending on the site of the injury, the nature and severity of trauma and the degree of secondary infection present. The most common variety of traumatic ulcer is single uncomplicated ulcer which generally is of moderate size

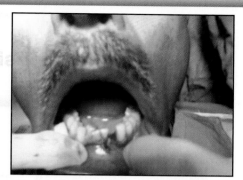

Fig. 8.1: Traumatic ulcer occurring in anterior region which is elliptical in shape

(from several millimeters to a centimeter or more in diameter), round, oval or elliptical in shape (Fig. 8.1) and flat or slightly depressed. Its surface consists of a serosanginous or grayish serofibronous exudate. It may be composed of a grayish necrotic slough which when removed, reveals a red raw tissue base. The lesion is surrounded by a narrow border of redness. There is tenderness and pain in the area of lesion and it will be helpful to identify the cause of lesion. In still other instances, the traumatic lesions are large and irregular. These are the result of unusually sever traumatic episodes, such as a blow or a fall and are often accompanied by considerable edema, inflammation and swelling of the neighboring tissues (Fig. 8.2). The infected ulcer is larger more irregular and more protruding than the non-infected one and often it is covered with a thick layer of necrotic slough through which purulent exudate may be observed.

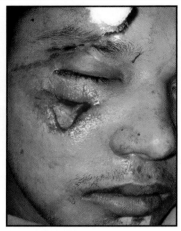

Fig. 8.2: Soft tissue ulcer occurring due to traumatic injury (*Courtesy:* Dr Lambade)

Usually the simple and uncomplicated traumatic ulcer heals uneventfully in 5 to 10 days after onset and even without treatment. However, in the presence of secondary infection or repetitive trauma longer healing period is required.

It is managed by remove of causative agent, anesthetic gel.

Drug Allergy

It is also called as 'drug idiosyncrasy', 'drug sensitivity' and 'stomatitis or dermatitis medicamentosa'. They may

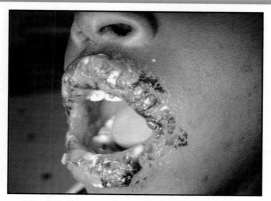

Fig. 8.3: Drug reaction occurring on lip showing extensive ulceration (*Courtesy*: Dr Revent Chole)

cause acute multiple ulcers and vesicles of oral mucosa or lichenoid reaction. Drugs which can most commonly cause drug reactions are aminopyrine, barbiturates, gold, bromide, penicillin, streptomycin, etc.

It is characterized by inflammation, ulceration and vesicle formation with arthralgia, fever and lymphadenopathy (Fig. 8.3). The skin lesion is often of erythematous type, as in erythema multiforme or they may be urticarial in nature. Fixed drug reaction - fixed drug reactions may occur in those who are administrated on repeated occasions, a drug to which they are sensitive. It consists of appearance of same reaction at the same site each time.

Orally the oral lesions are diffuse in distribution and vary in appearance from multiple areas of erythema to extensive areas of erosion or ulceration. In the early stages of reaction, vesicle or even bullae may be found on the mucosa. Occasionally purpuric spots appear and angioneurotic edema is seen.

The signs and symptoms of drug allergy regress with discontinuing of the causative drug. The acute signs may be relived by administration of antihistaminic drugs or cortisone.

Contact Allergy

It is caused by delayed type of hypersensitivity reaction to topical antigen. On the skin, it is referred as 'dermatitis venenata' and oral lesions are referred as 'stomatitis venenata'.

There are typically itching erythematous areas with superficial vesicle formation (Fig. 8.4), directly at the site

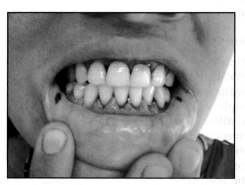

Fig. 8.4: Contact allergy occur due to dentifrices showing localized area of erythema (*Courtesy*: Dr Bhaskar Patle)

where allergen contacts skin. The skin may become thickened and dry. After the rupture of vesicle, erosion may become extensive and if secondary infection occurs, the lesion may be serious. Burning is a common complaint rather than itching of skin. Localized area of erythema, edema and vesiculation in specific areas of skin or mucosa whenever specific allergen is administered.

Oral lesions are rare due to number of Langerhans cells, saliva which dilutes the allergens and washes them from the surface of the mucosa and digest with enzymes and a thin layer of keratin present on the oral mucosa. Allergy to cinnamon oil or formalin present in tooth paste appears clinically as swelling, cracking and fissuring of lips, perioral desquamation and edema, angular cheilitis, swelling of gingiva and oral ulcerations.

Removal of allergen. Application of topical corticosteroids.

Angioneurotic Edema

It is also called as 'angioedema', 'Quincke's edema', 'and 'giant urticaria'. It is common form of edema occuring in both hereditary and non-hereditary forms. It is one form of acute anaphylactic reaction representing response allied to urticaria, allergic rhinitis and asthma.

The mechanism of development of swelling is due to vasodilation brought about by the release of histamine like substances with subsequent transudation of plasma.

Edema may develop gradually in a matter of hours, but can also progress in minutes. It typically manifests as a smooth, diffuse edematous swelling, particularly involving

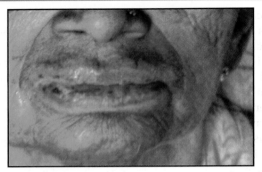

Fig. 8.5: Angioneurotic edema presented as swelling of lip appearing puffy (*Courtesy*: Dr Parate)

the face, around the lips (Fig. 8.5), chin and eyes, the tongue and sometimes, the hands and feet. Parotid gland may be affected in some cases. The eyes may be swollen, shut and lips may be extremely puffy. Symptoms may appear suddenly sometimes may present in morning. A feeling of tenderness or an itching or prickly sensation sometimes precedes the urticarial swelling.

When etiological agent such as food can be discovered, its elimination from diet will prevent recurrent attacks. Antihistaminic drugs (50 to 75 mg diphenylhydramine hydrochloride) can give prompt relief.

Aphthous Stomatitis

It is a common disease characterized by development of painful, recurrent, solitary or multiple ulcerations of the oral mucosa, with no other signs of any other disease.

It can be minor aphthae, major aphthae, herpetiform ulcers and recurrent ulcers associated with Behçet's syndrome.

It is caused by bacterial infection (a pleomorphic transitional L-form of α-hemolytic streptococcus and streptococcus sanguis), immunological abnormalities, iron deficiency or folic acid deficiency, hereditary, Hematological deficiency, serum iron or vitamin B_{12} deficiency, secondary malabsorption syndrome such as Celiac disease. It is precipitated by trauma, endocrine conditions, psychic factors, cessation of smoking and allergic factor.

It begins with prodormal burning for 24 to 48 hours, before the ulcer appears. It begins as a single or multiple superficial erosion covered by gray membrane. Localized areas of erythema develop and within hours small white papules form, ulcerate and gradually enlarge over next 48 to 72 hours. Lesions are round, symmetric and shallow but no tissue tags are present from the ruptured vesicles (Figs 8.6 and 8.7). The lesion is typically very painful so, it commonly interferes with eating for several days.

Minor aphthae: Size is 0.3 to 1 cm. Heal without scarring, within 10 to 14 days.

Major aphthae: Develop deep lesions, larger than 1 cm and may reach upto 5 cm in diameter. They interfere with speech and eating. Large portions may be covered with deep painful ulcers. The lesions heal slowly and leave scars, which result in decreased mobility of uvula and tongue and destruction of portions of oral mucosa (Fig. 8.8).

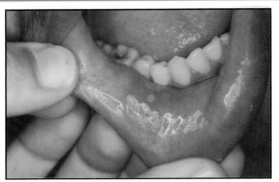

Fig. 8.6: Minor aphthous ulcer seen on lower lip presented with well-defined margin

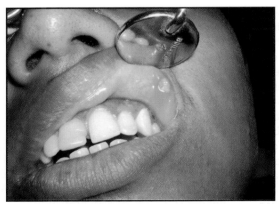

Fig. 8.7: Aphthous ulcer seen on upper lip

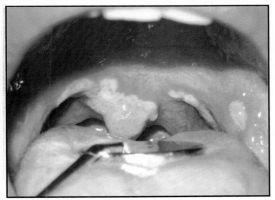

Fig. 8.8: Major aphthous ulcer on soft palate (*Courtesy*: Dr Soni)

Herpetiform ulcers: Multiple small shallow ulcers often up to 100 in number. Found on any intraoral mucosal surface. Begin as small pinhead size erosions that gradually enlarge and coalesce. Lesions are more painful than would be suspected by their size. Ulcer present continuously for one to three years, with relatively short remission. Patient gets relief immediately with 2 percent tetracycline mouthwash.

It is managed by topical protective emollient base (Orabase), topical tetracycline mouth wash (250 mg per ml) use four times daily for 5 to 7 days produces good response in nearly 70 percent of the patients, topical corticosteroid preparation- topical corticosteroid triamcinolone acetonide 3 to 4 times daily. In some severe cases fluocinolone gel, clobetasol cream or beclomethasone spray.

Erythema Multiforme

It is acute inflammatory disease of the skin and mucous membrane that causes a variety of skin lesions, hence the term 'multiforme'.

It can be self limiting form, severe form may be present as Steven-Johnson syndrome or toxic epidermal necrolysis and herpes associated erythema multiforme.

It is caused by immune mediated disease, drugs like sulfonamides, trimethoprin, nitrofurantion, phenylbutazone, digitalis, birth control pills and penicillin, microorganisms like mycoplasma pneumoniae and herpes simplex virus.

It has got acute or explosive onset with generalized symptoms such as fever and malaise. It may be asymptomatic and in less than 24 hours, extensive lesions of oral mucosa may appear. It is characterized by macule or papule, 0.5 to 2 cm in diameter, appearing in segmental distribution.

Bull's eye: Target or iris or bulls eye lesion consists of central bulla or pale clearing area, surrounded by edema and band of erythema.

Steven-Johnson syndrome: In Steven-Johnson syndrome, there is generalized vesicle and bulla formation involving skin, mouth, eyes and genitals.

Toxic epidermolysis necrolysis: It is also called as 'Lyell's disease'. It occurs secondary to drug reaction and results in sloughing of skin and mucosa in large sheets. It is managed in burn centers where necrotic skin is removed under general anesthesia and healing takes place under sheets of porcine xenografts.

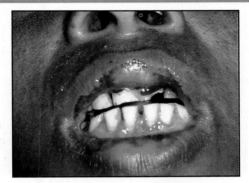

Fig. 8.9: Erythema multiforme showing
crusting of lip (*Courtesy*: Dr Bhaskar Patle)

Oral lesions start as bullae, on an erythematous base
and break rapidly into irregular ulcers. Patient cannot eat
or swallow and drools blood tinged saliva. The lesions are
larger, irregular, and deeper and often bleed very freely. In
full blown cases, lips are extensively involved (Figs 8.9 and
8.10) and large portions of the oral mucosa are denuded of
epithelium. Sloughing of mucosa and diffuse redness with
bright red raw surface is seen.

It is managed by 30 mg/day prednisolone or
methylprednisolone for several days and tapered after the
symptoms subside.

Pemphigus

It is autoimmune disease involving the skin and mucosa
and characterized by intraepidermal bulla formation.

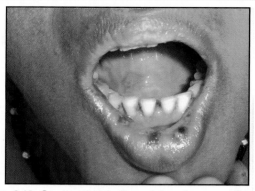

Fig. 8.10: Same patient in figure 8.9 erythema multiforme after treatment. (*Courtesy*: Dr Bhaskar Patle)

It can be pemphigus vulgaris, pemphigus vegetans, pemphigus foliaceous and pemphigus erythematosus.

Pemphigus vulgaris: Thin walled bullae or vesicles varying in diameter from few mm to several centimeters arise on normal skin or mucosa (Fig. 8.11). They rapidly break and continue to extend peripherally, eventually leaving large areas of denuded skin. After giving application of pressure to an intact bulla, the bulla will enlarge by extension to an apparently normal surfaces. Another characteristic sign of the disease is that pressure to an apparently normal area will result in formation of new lesion. This phenomenon is called as Nikolsky's sign. It is caused by prevesicular edema which disrupts the dermal-epidermal junctions. Oral lesions begin as classic bullae on non-inflamed base with formation

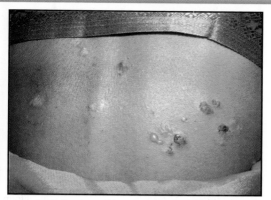

Fig 8.11: Intact vesicle seen on the back in patient
with pemphigus (*Courtesy*: Bhaskar Patle)

of shallow ulcers as bullae break rapidly. Thin layer of
epithelium peels away in an irregular pattern leaving
denuded base (Fig. 8.12). The lesion may have ragged
borders and be covered with white or blood tinged exudate.
Edges of the lesion may extend peripherally.

Pemphigus vegetans: It can be neumann type (early lesions
are similar to those seen in pemphigus vulgaris) and
hallopeau type (pustules, not bullae, are the initial lesions
which are followed by verrucous hyperkeratotic vegetations). The flaccid bullae become eroded and forms
'vegetations' on some of the erosions. The disease usually
terminates in pemphigus vulgaris. Gingival lesions may be
lace like ulcers with purulent surface on red base or have
granular or cobblestone appearance.

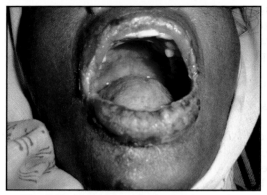

Fig. 8.12: Pemphigus vulgaris showing erosion
(*Courtesy*: Dr Revent Chole)

Pemphigus foliaceus: It is manifested by characteristic early bullous lesions which rapidly rupture and dry to leave masses of flakes on scales suggestive of an exfoliative dermatitis or eczema.

Brazilian pemphigus: It is a mild endemic form of pemphigus foliaceous found in tropical regions, particularly in Brazil. It is seen in children and frequently in family groups.

Pemphigus erythematosus: It is form of disease which is characterized by the occurrence of bullae and vesicles concomitant with the appearance of crusted patches resembling seborrheic dermatitis or even lupus erythematosus. Most cases ultimately terminate in pemphigus vulgaris or foliaceous. The skin manifestations in any form of pemphigus may be accompanied by fever and malaise.

It is managed by corticosteroids, plasmapheresis, parenteral gold therapy, etretinate and dapsone and administration of 8-methoxypsoralen, followed by exposure of peripheral blood to ultraviolet radiation.

Bullous Pemphigoid

It is also called as 'para-pemphigus', or 'aging pemphigus'. In this, the initial defect is sub-epithelial in the lamina lucida region of the basement membrane. It is associated with anti-basement membrane antibodies which are detected in the basement membrane.

Bullae do not extend peripherally and remain localized; heal spontaneously. Skin lesions begin as generalized non-specific rash, commonly on the limbs, which appear as blisters on inflamed skin; itching precedes. These vesicle and bullae are relatively thick walled and may remain intact for some days.

Oral lesions are smaller, form more slowly and are less painful. Gingival lesions consist of generalized edema, inflammation, desquamation and localized areas of discrete vesicle formation. Vesicles and ultimately erosion may develop not only on the gingival tissue but any other area such as the buccal mucosa, palate, floor of the mouth and tongue (Fig. 8.13).

It is managed by systemic steroids in lower doses, for shorter period combined with immunosuppressive drugs and Dapsone.

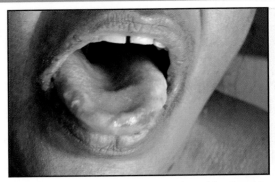

Fig. 8.13: Vesicle and with erosion seen on lateral border of tongue in patient with bullous pemphigoid (*Courtesy*: Dr Revent Chole)

Benign Mucous Membrane Pemphigoid

It is also called as 'cicatrical pemphigoid'. It is a disease of unknown etiology but probably is autoimmune in nature.

Adhesions may develop between bulbar and palpebral conjunctivae resulting in obliteration of the palpebral fissure leading to blindness. Involvement of esophagus and trachea may cause strictures leading to difficulty in swallowing or breathing. It may lead to scarring of affected area.

The mucosal lesions are also vesiculobullous in nature, but appear to be relatively thick walled and for this reason may persist for 24 to 48 hours before rupturing and desquamation. After rupture of vesicle surface epithelium is lost leaving raw red bleeding surface. Gingiva is edematous and bright red, involvement is patchy and

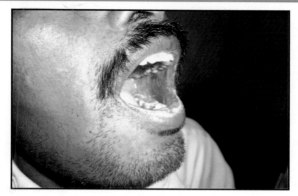

Fig. 8.14: Cicatrical pemphigoid showing erosion of cheek (*Courtesy*: Dr Revent Chole)

diffuse. There may be formation of ulcer, which surrounded by zone of erythema. There may be erosion on cheek (Fig. 8.14) and vesicles on palate and narrower peripheral extensions.

Topical and intralesional steroids, dapsone therapy, systemic steroids and immunosuppressive therapy.

Familial Benign Chronic Pemphigus

It is also called as Hailey-Hailey disease. It is uncommon disease transmitted by irregular dominant gene.

Heat and sweating amplify the outbreak of the lesion while spontaneous remission may occur in cold weather. The lesions develop as small groups of vesicles appearing on normal or erythematous skin, which soon rupture to

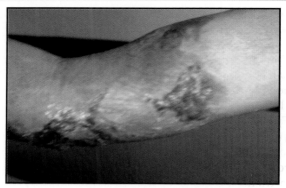

Fig. 8.15: Familial chronic pemphigus showing eroded surface hand (*Courtesy*: Dr Tapasya)

leave eroded, crusted areas (Fig. 8.15). Nikolsky's sign - they enlarge peripherally but heal in center with Nikolsky's sign positive. Tender and enlarged regional lymph nodes may also be present.

Oral lesions are similar to those occurring on the skin and it develops as crops of vesicle, which rapidly ruptures leaving raw eroded areas.

Antibiotics therapy is generally effective in this lesion.

Epidermolysis Bullosa

It is a dermatological disorder in which bullae or vesicles occur on skin or mucous membrane surface spontaneously, shortly after minor trauma. It can be epidermolysis bullosa simplex, epidermolysis bullosa dystrophic, dominant, epidermolysis bullosa dystrophic, recessive, functional epidermolysis bullosa and epidermolysis bullosa acquista (acquired).

Epidermolysis bullosa simplex - it is characterized by formation of bullae or vesicle on the hands and feet at site of friction or trauma. The knees, elbows and trunk are rarely involved and nails are occasionally affected.

Epidermolysis bullosa dystrophic dominant - hair may be sparse, while nails are usually dystrophic or absent with milia present. Palmar-planter keratoderma with hyperhidrosis also may occur with ichthyosis and sometimes hypertrichosis.

Epidermolysis bullosa dystrophic recessive - Nikolsky's sign is positive in this type of epidermolysis bullosa. The bullae contain a clear, bacteriologically sterile or sometime blood tinged fluid. When these bullae rupture or are peeled off under trauma or pressure, they leave raw, painful surface (Fig. 8.16). The bullae heal by scar and milia formation which may result in afunctional club-like fists. The hair may be sparse (Fig. 8.17), while the nails are usually dystrophic (Fig. 8.18).

Junctional epidermolysis bullosa - it is extremely sever form of the dystrophic recessive form, which is incompatible with prolonged survival. It has onset at birth, absence of scarring, milia, pigmentation and death within three months of age. The bullae are similar to recessive form but they develop simultaneously and sheets of skin may actually be shed.

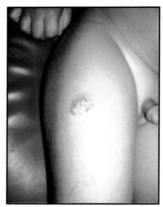

Fig. 8.16: Vesicle formation seen on leg at contact area in patient of epidermolysis bullosa

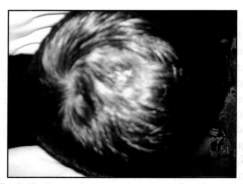

Fig. 8.17: Sparse hair seen in patient of epidermolysis bullosa. Also note vesicle in the scalp

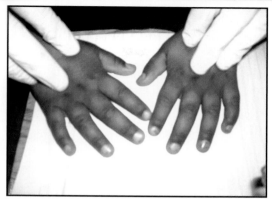

Fig. 8.18: Dystrophic nails seen in patient of epidermolysis bullosa

Oral lesion more commonly seen in recessive type. These bullae are painful especially when they rupture or when the epithelium desquamates (Fig. 8.19). Scar formation results in obliteration of sulci and restriction of the tongue movement. Hoarseness and dysphagia may occur as a result of bullae of larynx and pharynx. Esophageal involvement produces serious strictures. Dental defects like rudimentary teeth, congenitally absent teeth, hypoplastic teeth and crowns denuded of enamel may be seen.

Large blisters should be pricked and the blister fluid released. Dressing, to minimize reaction may be helpful. Super infections should be treated with appropriate local or systemic antibiotics.

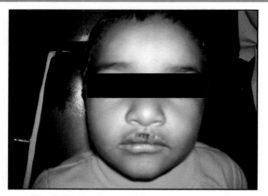

Fig. 8.19: Rupture vesicle seen on upper lip

Steven-Johnson Syndrome

It is the severe form of erythema multiforme with widespread involvement, typically involving skin, oral cavity, eyes and genitalia.

It commences with abrupt occurrence of fever, malaise, photophobia and eruptions on oral mucosa, genital mucosa and skin.

Cutaneous lesions: Cutaneous lesions are similar to erythema multiforme and are hemorrhagic, often vesicular or bullous.

Eye lesions: It consists of photophobia, conjunctivitis, corneal ulcerations. Keratoconjunctivitis sicca has also been described and blindness may result, chiefly from intercurrent bacterial infection.

Genital lesions: Genital lesions are reported to consist of non-specific urethritis, balanitis and vaginal ulcers.

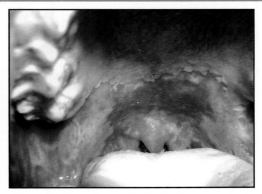

Fig. 8.20: Extensive oral lesion in Steven-Johnson syndrome (*Courtesy*: Dr Parate)

Complications: Other reported complications are related to respiratory tract involvement such as tracheo-bronchial ulcerations and pneumonia.

Oral mucous membrane lesions may be extremely painful and so, mastication becomes impossible. Mucosal vesicles or bullae occur, rupture and leave a surface covered with a thick, white or yellow exudate (Fig. 8.20). Lips may exhibit ulcerations with bloody crusting and are often painful.

There is no specific treatment for this, although in some cases, ACTH, cortisone and chlortetracycline have shown promising results.

Oral Ulcers Secondary to Cancer Chemotherapy

It may be due to direct effect on replication and growth of oral epithelium by interfering with nucleic acid and protein

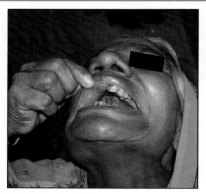

Fig. 8.21: Oral ulceration seen in patient who is receiving chemotherapy

synthesis and leading to thinning and ulceration of oral mucosa, e.g. by methotrexate.

Alopecia occur due to arrest of mitosis of the rapidly germinating hair root. Stomatitis occurs with diffuse (Fig. 8.21) inflammatory changes developed in mucosa. Distinct blebs or whitish areas result from decreased cellular division and retention of squamous cells. There is also burning sensation in the oral cavity with mucosal erosion. In subse-quent weeks, surface layer is lost and thin erythematous mucosa is present. Focal areas ulcerate and then become covered with tan yellow fibrous exudate.

Topical anesthetic such as elixir of diphenhydramine or lidocaine combined with milk of magnesia. Oral suspension of tetracycline which is used as mouth washes and then swallowed.

Infection of
Oral Cavity

PERIAPICAL OSTEITIS

Microorganisms responsible for deep carious lesions penetrate the pulp and stimulate inflammation within soft pulpal tissue, ultimately leading to necrosis of pulp. The bacteria from necrotic pulp invade the marrow spaces of bone in the periapical region and trigger the process of inflammation. This stage is called as periapical osteitis.

The later consequences are edema (Fig. 9.1), ischemia and necrosis. The path of least resistance is along medullary spaces. The patient gets throbbing pain and there is marked tenderness to vertical percussion. Clinician should prefer either endodontic treatment or extraction of tooth, under antibiotic coverage. Antibiotics should be continued for three to five days after extraction.

Cellulitis

It is also called 'Phlegmon'. Occasionally, the infectious process progresses out of the bone, despite the use of supportive therapy and the patient develops cellulites, either in vestibular region or extraorally. It is a potential complication of acute dental infection.

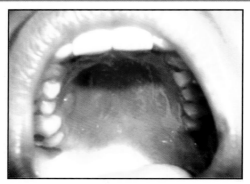

Fig. 9.1: Periapical osteitis showing swelling in the periapical area

Cellulitis is defined as a non-suppurative inflammation of the subcutaneous tissues extending along the connective tissue planes and across the intercellular spaces.

There is widespread swelling, redness and pain without definite localization. Presence of tenderness on palpation. Tissues are grossly edematous (Fig. 9.2). There is marked induration; hence tissues are firm to hard on palpation. Tissues are often discolored; temperature is elevated with malaise and lethargy. Usually massive cellulitis will ultimately suppurate, particularly if bacteria are staphylococcal. Depending upon the location and proximity to anatomic structures that guide the progress, the pus may evacuate into nose, maxillary sinus, oral vestibule, floor of mouth, infratemporal fossa and into fascial spaces.

It is managed by surgical incision and drainage.

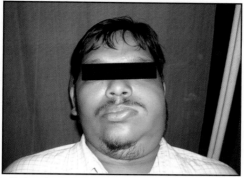

Fig. 9.2: Patient having cellulitis showing swelling on left side face which involving submandibular space, pterygomandibular space

Acute Periapical Abscess

It is also called as 'acute alveolar abscess'. It is a localized collection of pus in the alveolar bone, at the root apex of a tooth, following death of the pulp.

It may be result of trauma or chemical or mechanical irritation. The immediate cause is the bacterial invasion of dead pulp. When inflammatory response extend into adjacent periapical alveolar bone, it will initiate necrosis of periapical tissue and diffuse rarefaction of bone, leading to formation of periapical abscess with symptoms of acute inflammation.

Pain is severe and of throbbing type. Patients experience sensitivity or pressure in the affected area. Ice relives the pain and heat intensifies it. Aspiration yield yellowish pus. The tooth becomes more painful, appears elongated and

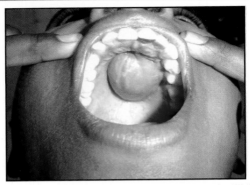

Fig. 9.3: Periapical abscess seen on the palate (*Courtesy:* Dr Bhaskar Patle, Lecturer, Oral Medicine and Radiology, SPDC Wardha, India)

mobile. In acute periapical infection, tooth is sensitive to percussion and movement. There is also painful lymphadenopathy. After some period the affected pulp is necrotic and does not respond to electric current or to application of cold. Swelling is usually seen in adjacent tissues adjacent to the affected tooth (Fig. 9.3). The tissues at the surface of swelling appear taut and inflamed. The surface of tissue become distended from the pressure of underlying pus and finally ruptures due to pressure and lack of resistance caused by continued liquefaction.

Radiologically, swelling of periodontal ligament space force the tooth slightly from its socket, creating widening of periodontal ligament space (Fig. 9.4). After some period the first change is usually of slight unsharpness of some of the trabeculae at the tooth apex.

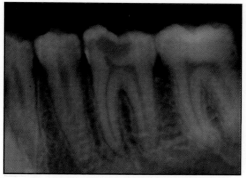

Fig. 9.4: Acute apical periodontitis presented as PDL space widening in relation with first molar (*Courtesy:* Dr Ashok L, Professor and Head, Oral Medicine and Radiology, Bapuji Dental College and Hospital, Davanagere, India)

It is managed by drainage; antibiotics like penicillin 500 mg, QID, for 5 days and analgesics should be given. If there is need of retention of offending tooth, necrotic pulp should be extirpated and tooth should be treated endodontically.

Periodontal Abscess

It is usually culmination of a long period of chronic periodontitis. It usually occurs in pre-existing periodontal pocket. When such pocket reaches sufficient depth of about 5 to 8 mm, the soft tissues, around the neck of the tooth may approximate the tooth so tightly that orifice of the pocket is occluded. Bacteria multiply in the depth of pocket and cause sufficient irritation to form an acute abscess, with exudation of pus into this area.

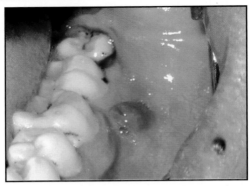

Fig. 9.5: Periodontal infection showing a swelling over the root surface

It starts at the gingival crevice and extends down on one or more surface of the root, frequently as far as apical region. Acute episode usually has sudden onset with extreme pain. There is also distension and discomfort. They are associated with swelling of the soft tissues overlying the surface of the involved root (Fig. 9.5). Tooth is tender and mobile. Pus usually exudes from the gingival crevice.

Primary treatment for relief of acute symptoms is incision of the fluctuant abscess, from the depth of the abscess cavity to the gingiva.

Acute Exacerbation of a Chronic Lesion

It is also called as 'phoenix abscess.' It is an acute inflammatory reaction superimposed on an existing chronic lesion, such as on cyst or granuloma.

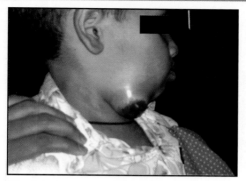

Fig. 9.6: Acute exacerbation of chronic infection swelling due to hot fomentation

The periradicular area may react to noxious stimuli from a diseased pulp with chronic periradicular disease. At times, because of an influx of necrotic product from a diseased pulp or because of bacteria and there toxins, this apparently dormant lesion may react and cause an acute inflammatory response.

At the onset, tooth may be tender to touch. Patients complain of intense pain, local swelling and possibly associated cellulitis. Mucosa over the radicular area may be sensitive to palpation and may appear red and swollen (Fig. 9.6). Lack of response to vitality test points to diagnosis necrotic pulp.

Radiologically, there may be radiolucency or rarefaction at the apex (Fig. 9.7).

Drainage, either via the root canal or by incision, if there is localized swelling.

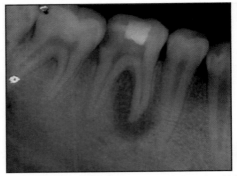

Fig. 9.7: Periapical rarefaction in case of phoenix abscess

Pericoronal Abscess

It is also called as 'pericoronitis'. It is the infection of soft tissues surrounding the crown of a partially erupted tooth.

The most common type of pericoronal infection is found around the mandibular 3rd molar.

It may result in cellulitis and muscular trismus. There is also regional lymphadenopathy, submaxillary and pharyngeal abscess. Operculum may get traumatized by opposing teeth during mastication (Fig. 9.8). Edema, visible in both submandibular area and peritonsillar region. There is extreme tenderness on palpation of the abscess. Pain, malaise and swelling of peritonsillar region.

Radiologically defect in bone on mesial or distal (Fig. 9.9) side which appears as the step like distortion of crypt wall distal to the crown. In cases of lower third molar, there is circumferential bone resorption around the tooth.

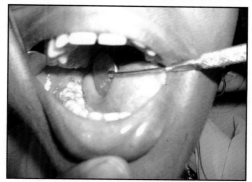

Fig. 9.8: Pericoronitis seen as flap on the third molar with inflammation

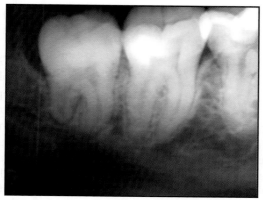

Fig. 9.9: Distal bone loss seen in relationship with 3rd molar

Most commonly used antibiotics are phenoxylmethyl penicillin 250 mg four times daily. In pericoronitis due to ulceromembranous gingivitis metronidazole 200 gm three times daily for 7 days is given. Operculectomy - sometimes when the retention of 3rd molar is necessary, the inflamed tissue surrounding the occlusal portion of the tooth should be excided.

Ludwig's Angina

It is a condition which was first described by Ludwig in 1936. The word angina means sensation of choking or suffocation. It is the most commonly encountered neck space infection. This condition may be defined as an over-whelming, rapidly spreading, septic cellulitis involving submandibular, submental and sublingual spaces bilaterally.

It is caused by odontogenic infection, trauma, sialadenitis, calculi, and osteomyelitis.

It is characterized by brawny indurations. Tissues are board like and do not pit on pressure. No fluctuance is present. The tissues may become gangrenous and when cut, they have a peculiar lifeless appearance. A sharp limitation is present between the infected tissues and surrounding normal tissues. Three facial spaces are involved bilaterally, i.e. submandibular, submental and sublingual. If the involvement is not bilateral, the infection is not considered a typical Ludwig's angina.

The mouth is open (Fig. 9.10) and the tongue is lifted upwards and backwards, so that it is pushed against the

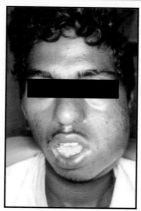

Fig. 9.10: Ludwig angina showing open mouth appearance

roof of the mouth and the posterior pharyngeal wall; when this occurs, acute respiratory obstruction is likely to occur. On CT air filled cavity can be seen.

It is managed by intense and prolonged antibiotic therapy; establishment and maintenance of an adequate airway are the essentials of therapy, incision and drainage and supportive therapy (parenteral hydration, high protein diet and vitamin supplements).

Chronic Alveolar Abscess

It is a long standing, low grade infection of the periradicular tissues.

It results from direct extension of acute pulpitis or acute non-suppurative periodontitis or acute exacerbation of periapical granuloma, cyst or chronic abscess. The surrounding tissue attempt to localize the pyogenic infection by forming enclosure of granulation tissue; this in turn is surrounded by fibrous connective tissue; this results in well circumscribed lesion containing necrotic tissue.

It is characterized by less soreness and often, a better defined radiographic lesion. Tooth is tender, vitality test is negative. Draining fistulas are also commonly associated with chronic alveolar abscess (Fig. 9.11). The patients will demonstrate lymphadenopathy as well.

Radiologically there is loss of thickness and density of the apical portion of lamina dura of the affected tooth.

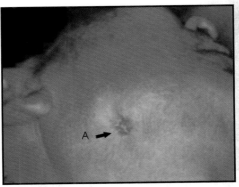

Fig. 9.11: Chronic infection showing extraoral sinus

Widespread area of diffuse demineralization of the periapical bone, of affected tooth becomes apparent (Fig. 9.12). Margins vary from well-defined with possible hyperostotic borders to poorly defined, in chronic cases (Fig. 9.13). After some period, the trabeculae which are rarefied are destroyed and the dark area become darker and larger, as more of the surrounding bone is taken into the diseased area.

If there is need of retention of offending tooth, necrotic pulp should be opened and tooth should be treated endodontically.

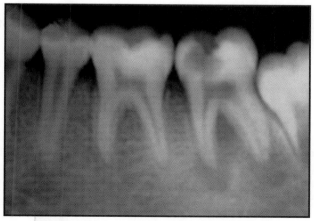

Fig. 9.12: Severe caries in relations with second molar which also show periapical radiolucency

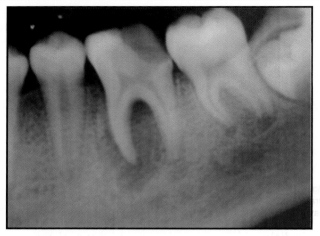

Fig. 9.13: Periapical rarefaction seen as decreased radiodensity in relation with first molar

Condensing Osteitis

It is also called as 'chronic focal sclerosing osteo-myelitis'. If the exudate is of low toxicity and long standing then the resulting mild irritation may lead to circumscribed proli-feration of periapical bone, appearing as condensing osteitis or focal sclerosing osteomyelitis. There is deposition of new bone along the existing trabeculae, a process knows as appositional bone deposition.

Tooth is usually asymptomatic. But in some cases, patient may report pain or tenderness on percussion or palpation.

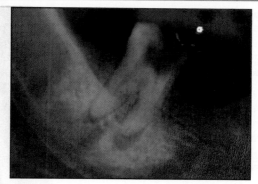

Fig. 9.14: Condensing osteitis (*Courtesy:* Dr Ashok L, Professor and Head, Oral Medicine and Radiology, Bapuji Dental College and Hospital, Davanagere, India)

Radiologically it appears as localized area of radiopacity surrounding the affected tooth, which may extend below the apex (Fig. 9.14). It may be variable in size and extent, with margins from well defined to very diffuse. At the diffused margins, the thickened trabeculae can be seen in continuation of adjacent normal bone.

Periapical Granuloma

It is the most common type of pathologic radiolucency encountered in dentistry.

The tooth is non-vital, i.e. it does not respond to thermal and electric pulp test. Tooth may be darker in color, because of the blood pigments that diffuse into the dentinal tubules. Mild pain can be occasionally experienced while biting or chewing on solid foods. Sensitivity occurs due to hyperemia, edema and inflammation of the apical periodontal ligament.

Radiologically periapical area is radiolucent with loss of lamina dura. Radiolucency is less than 1.5 cm in diameter (Fig. 9.15). There may or may not be hyperostotic borders. It may or may not have well defined borders.

Extraction of the involved tooth or under certain conditions, root canal therapy, with or without subsequent apicoectomy are the treatment options.

Osteomyelitis

It is the inflammation of the bone marrow that produces clinically apparent pus and secondarily affects the calcified

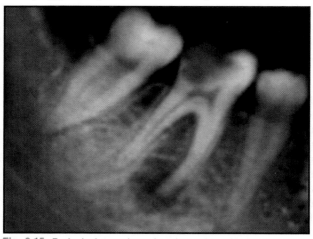

Fig. 9.15: Periapical granuloma in relationship with the first molar

components. It is infection of the bone that involves all the three components viz. periosteum, cortex and marrow. It may be defined as an inflammatory condition of the bone that begins as an infection of medullary cavity and the haversian system and extends to involve the periosteum of the affected area.

It is predisposed by diabetes mellitus, tuberculosis, severe anemia, leukemia, agranulocytosis, acute illness such as influenza, scarlet fever, typhoid and exanthematous fever, sickle cell anemia, malnutrition and chronic alcoholism.

It is caused odontogenic infections, compound fractures of the jaws, traumatic injury, middle ear infection and respiratory infection, furunculosis of chin, and peritonsillar abscess.

It can be acute suppurative osteomyelitis, chronic suppurative osteomyelitis, infantile osteomyelitis, chronic non-suppurative, radiation osteomyelitis, Garre's osteomyelitis.

Acute suppurative osteomyelitis—It is serious sequelae of periapical infection there is often a diffuse spread of infection throughout the medullary spaces, with subsequent necrosis of variable amount of bone (Figs 9.16 and 9.17). It has rapid onset and course, severe pain, paresthesia or anesthesia of the mental nerve. Pus exudates around the gingival sulcus or through mucosal and cutaneous fistula. Firm cellulitis of cheek and abscess formation with localized warmth and tenderness on palpation. The patient feels toxic and dehydrated. Radiologically about 10 days after acute infection, the density of trabeculae will be decreased and

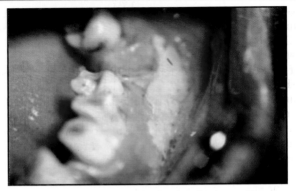

Fig. 9.16: Osteomyelitis showing dead necrotic bone in the mandible

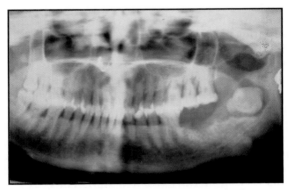

Fig. 9.17: OPG showing radiopaque dead necrotic bone on left side of mandible in ramus

become blurred and fuzzy. There is loss of continuity of lamina dura, which is seen in more than one tooth.

Chronic suppurative osteomyelitis—Chronic osteomyelitis develops without initial acute stage, if the virulence is of low grade. Chronic osteomyelitis is persistent abscess of the bone that is characterized by usual complex inflammatory process including necrosis of mineralized and marrow tissues, suppuration, resorption sclerosis and hyperplasia. Local tenderness and swelling develop over the bone in the area of abscess. Intraorally and extraorally sinus develops intermittently and drains small amount of pus and then gradually heals. Painless unless there is an acute or subacute exacerbation.

Radiologically single or multiple radiolucencies of variable size. Irregular outline and poorly defined borders (Fig. 9.18). 'Moth eaten appearances' is seen as the radiolucent areas enlarge and become irregular in outline and get separated by islands of normal appearing bone (Fig. 9.19). This is due to the enlargement of medullary spaces and widening of Volkmann's canals, secondary to lysis of bone and replacement with granulation tissue. Segments of necrotic bone become detached; irregular calcified areas separate from the remaining bone and become distinguishable as sequestra. Sequestra are more dense and better defined due to following reasons (Fig. 9.20) Sclerosis that was induced before the bone became necrotic. Dead bone has affinity for calcium. Hence, it absorbs calcium. In patients with extensive chronic osteomyelitis, the disease may spread to mandibular condyle and joint, resulting in septic arthritis.

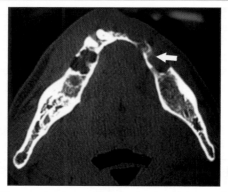

Fig. 9.18: CT scan of osteomyelitis showing bone destruction (*Courtesy:* Dr Chandrasekhar Bande, Lecturer, Oral and Maxillofacial Surgery, GDCH, Nagpur, India)

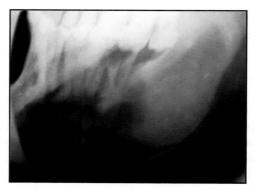

Fig. 9.19: Osteomyelitis with pathological fracture in body of mandible

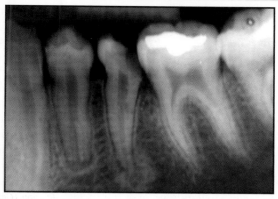

Fig. 9.20: Focal sclerosing osteomyelitis (*Courtesy:* Dr Ashok L, Professor and Head, Oral Medicine and Radiology. Bapuji Dental College and Hospital, Davanagere, India)

Sclerosing osteomyelitis - reactive proliferation of bone is the primary response in diffuse sclerosing osteomyelitis due to a balance between the virulence of infection and resistance of host. It is analogous to focal form of the disease. It occurs due to low grade infection. Symptoms are very mild or absent. During the period of growth the patient complains of pain and tenderness. Pain persists for few weeks to months to even years. Jaws may be slightly enlarged on the affected side. Radiologically there is presence of osteolytic and osteosclerotic zones. As the lesion progresses there is increase in the size of the involved part. Margins are ill-defined.

Garre's osteomyelitis—It is also called as 'proli-ferative periostitis. It is characterized by formation of hard bony swelling at the periphery of the jaw. For the lesion to develop following conditions should be satisfied. The periosteum must possess high potential for osteoblastic activity. Mild infection serves as a stimulus. Fine balance should be maintained between the resistance of host and number and virulence of organisms. It is presented as hard non-tender swelling with medial and lateral expansion of jaw. There is also lymphadenopathy; hyperpyrexia and leukocytosis are common findings. Radiologically intraoral radiograph will reveal a carious tooth opposite the hard bony mass. Shadow of thin convex shell of bone over the cortex may be seen. No trabecular pattern between shell of new bone and cortex. As infection persists, the cortex thickens and becomes lami-nated with alternating radiopaque and radiolucent layers (onion peel (skin) appearances).

It is managed by incision and drainage, irrigation and debridment of the necrotic areas, antibiotics, extraction of offending tooth, adequate rehydration, rich nutritional diet, multivitamin, sequestrectomy, saucerization, decortication, and hyperbaric oxygen therapy.

Facial Space Infections

Facial spaces are potential spaces situated between the planes of fascia, which form natural pathways along which the infection may spread (Fig. 9.21).

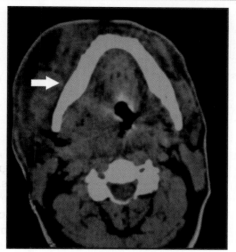

Fig. 9.21: Facial space infection presenting as air cavity on CT scan (*Courtesy:* Dr Datarkar, Asso. Professor, Oral and Maxillofacial Surgery, SPDC, Wardha, India)

Canine Space

Swelling just lateral to the nose, obliterating the nasolabial fold. Intraorally, swelling is present in the labial sulcus (Fig. 9.22). Rarely, palatal swelling is encountered.

Buccal Space

Maxillary and mandibular molar or premolar, if apex is above the attachment. Facial swelling with little trismus.

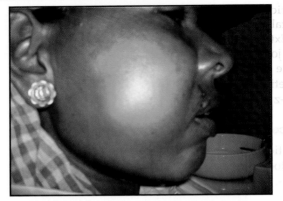

Fig. 9.22: Canine space infection which also involve buccal space seen as huge swelling

Parotid Space

It reaches from the lateral pharyngeal space or by retrograde extension along the parotid gland.

The swelling extends from the level of the zygomatic arch to the lower border of the mandible. Posteriorly, it extends into the retromandibular region and anteriorly, it ends at the end of the anterior border of ramus. The swelling tends to evert the lobule of ear.

Infratemporal Space

Infratemporal infection can extend via the plexus of veins, through the inferior orbital fissure into the terminal part of inferior ophthalmic vein and then, through the superior orbital fissure into cavernous sinus.

Extraoral swelling over the region of sigmoid notch and TMJ joint area (Fig. 9.23) and intraorally swelling is usually in the tuberosity area. The patient may exhibit trismus and sometimes swelling of eyelids, if there is involvement of post-zygomatic fossa.

Space for the Body of Mandible

Infection may arise from fracture or by direct extension from the floor of mouth, lateral pharyngeal spaces and masticator space. Infection may be dental, periodontal or vascular in origin.

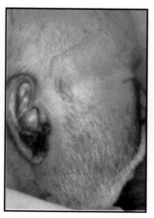

Fig. 9.23: Infratemporal space infection seen as as swelling on TMJ area (*Courtesy:* Dr Lambade)

There is induration or fluctuation of the labial sulcus, if the outer cortical plate is involved. When the inner cortical plate is involved, the infection is restricted to the floor of mouth.

Submental Space

Chin becomes grossly swollen, quiet firm and erythematous (Fig. 9.24). Slight extraoral swelling just below the chin is evident.

Submandibular Space

It originates from the mandibular molars. Carious mandibular molar is usually present. It produces a swelling

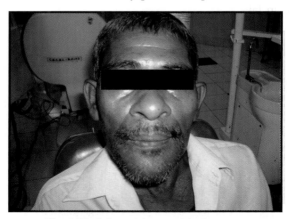

Fig. 9.24: Submental space infection seen showing grossly swollen chin

near the angle of the jaw, which is brawny edematous in appearance (Fig. 9.25). After some days, swelling becomes soft and fluctuant. Because of anatomic proximity, there is usually involvement of glands and nodes, resulting in sialadenitis and lymphadenitis.

Sublingual Space

The infection may arise directly from perforation of the lingual cortical plate, above the mylohyoid attachment or by extension from other spaces, primarily submandibular space.

Brawny erythematous tender swelling of the floor of mouth is present. Swelling is close to mandible and spreads towards midline or beyond. Elevation of the tongue may be noted in late cases.

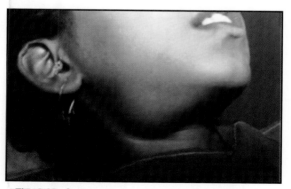

Fig. 9.25: Submandibular space infection presented as swelling in the submandibular area

Masticator Space

The swelling may be either external or internal, or both. The external swelling consists of brawny induration over the ramus and angle of mandible (Fig. 9.26). Internal swelling may predominate in some cases. Such swelling involves the sublingual region and the pharyngeal wall.

The pharyngeal swelling pushes palatine tonsils towards midline. Pain is excruciating and often radiates to the ear. Dysphagia may be present, especially when the swelling is internal. Clinically masticatory space infection is likely to be marked by severe trismus because of irritation of masseter and medial pterygoid. It can be so severe that the mouth opening is restricted only to half a centimeter.

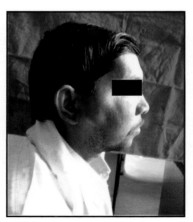

Fig. 9.26: Submasseteric space infection showing swelling over the ramus and TMJ area

Temporal Space

In case of infection with superficial temporal space, swelling is limited below by the zygomatic arch and laterally, it is limited by the outline of superficial and temporal line. Due to limited distention of temporal facia, the pain is severe. A deep temporal abscess produces less swelling than one involving the superficial temporal space.

Pterygomandibular Space

There is no external evidence of swelling. Intraoral examination reveals an anterior bulging of half of the soft palate. Deviation of tongue to the affected side. Severe trismus and difficulty in swallowing. It must be distinguished from peritonsillar abscess. In latter, there is no offending tooth and trismus is less severe.

FATAL COMPLICATIONS OF ORAL INFECTION

Bacterial Meningitis

It is the most common neurologic complication resulting from oral and maxillofacial infections. In this condition bacteria infect arachnoid pia mater and CSF. The infection quickly spreads from its point of origin, via CSF, to the entire subarachnoid space.

Headache, chills, fever and nausea. Pain in back and stiffness of neck. Kernig's and Brudzinski's signs are positive, seizures, confusion and stupor. Diagnosis is made by lumbar puncture and CSF examination.

It is a medical emergency and prompt intravenous antibiotics should be started, after antibiotic sensitivity testing.

Cavernous Sinus Thrombosis

It is one of the most dreaded and life-threatening complication due to intracranial spread of infection from odontogenic source.

The bacteria can reach cavernous sinus in septic emboli through venous and arterial systems. Septic thrombophlebitis of emmissary veins can directly lead to this phenomenon.

Eye: Proptosis or protrusion of eye is seen as a result of decreased venous drainage, chemosis and edema of eyelid, which is secondary to venous stasis.

Cranial nerve involvement: Limitation of extraocular movements because of involvement of 3rd, 4th and 6th cranial nerves.

Massive doses of antibiotics, with proper surgical intervention at the primary site of infection are essential.

Odontogenic Infection of Orbit

Odontogenic infection can spread to orbit through several routes. Infection of premolars and molars can perforate the maxillary buccal plate and can spread to pterygopalatine and infra-temporal fossa and reach the orbit, via inferior orbital fissure. The maxillary anterior teeth can produce orbital cellulitis (Fig. 9.27) by retrograde spread through vessels like anterior facial, angular and ophthalmic vein.

It can result in significant morbidity and mortality. It may result in temporary loss of visual acuity.

Necrotizing Fasciitis

This condition was first recognized in 1924 by Meleney. It is defined as rapidly progressing necrosis of subcutaneous tissue and fascia, usually sparing the muscles and accompanied by toxicity, high fever and apathy.

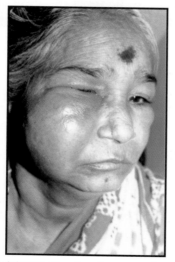

Fig. 9.27: Infection of oral cavity can reach to the orbit

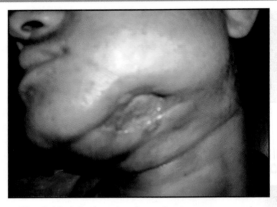

Fig. 9.28: Infection showing subcutaneous necrosis
in case of necrotizing fasciitis

A tender erythematous cellulitis with ill-defined margins presents the patient with high fever and apathy. Pain can be severe. There is paresthesia of affected skin, secondary to cutaneous nerve destruction, which can occur before clinical gangrene. Skin bullae may develop, but lymph adenitis is usually not seen. Skin death subsequent to subcutaneous necrosis is common (Fig. 9.28).

Spectrum of antibiotics should include drugs active against anaerobic organisms such as metronidazole. Continuous wound care is of utmost important. Hyperbaric oxygen therapy has been used, but its value is not proven.

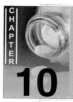

Oral Pigmentation

CLINICAL CLASSIFICATION ACCORDING TO COLOR

Color	Focal	Diffuse	Multifocal
Blue/ purple	Varix, Hemangioma	Hemangioma	Kaposi's sarcoma, Hereditary hemorrhagic telangiectasia
Brown	Melanotic macules, nevus, melanoma	Ecchymosis, melanoma, drug induced, hairy tongue, petechiae	Physiologic pigmentation, neurofibromatosis, lichen planus, Addison's disease, drug induced, Peutz-Jeghers syndrome
Grey black	Amalgam tattoo, graphite tattoo, nevus, melanoma	Amalgam tattoo, hairy tongue	Metal ingestion

BLUE/PURPLE VASCULAR LESIONS

Hemangioma

It may be any congenital and traumatic in origin. It is characterized by proliferation of blood vessels.

Depending upon the depth of vascular proliferation within oral submucosa, the lesion may harbor vessels close to the overlying epithelium and appear *reddish blue* (Fig. 10.1) or if in the connective tissue, it will appear *blue* (Fig. 10.2). It may appear as a *flat reddish blue* macule (port wine stain) to a nodular blue tumefaction.

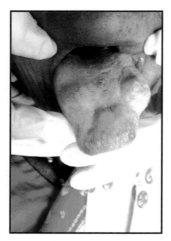

Fig. 10.1: Hemangioma of the showing reddish blue pigmentation

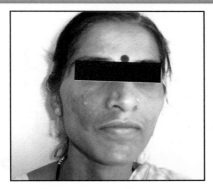

Fig. 10.2: Port wine stain present on right side of face as a flat reddish macule

VARICES AND VARIX

It is distended vein which may result from partial blockage of vein.

Varices

Pathological dilatation of vein or venules are varices or varicosity. Ventral surface of the tongue is chief site of involvement (Fig. 10.3). They appear as tortuous serpentine, blue red or purple elevations. They are painless and not subjected to rupture or hemorrhage.

Varix

Focal dilatation of group of venules or vein is known as varix. Primarily located on lower lip. The typical location of

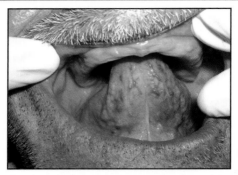

Fig. 10.3: Varices seen on ventral surface of the
tongue appearing as purple elevation

varix is in areas prone to pinching trauma. It is usually
small in diameter ranging from 2-4 mm. It appears as blue,
red or purple raised pigmentation often lobulated or
nodular. It has sharply delineated borders and a smooth,
rounded surface contour.

The lesion can be excised or removed by electrosurgery
or cryosurgery.

ANGIOSARCOMA

It is a malignant vascular neoplasm in the oral cavity. They
are rapidly proliferative and therefore present as nodular
tumors. If superficial, it appears as red, blue or purple
nodular tumor.

KAPOSI'S SARCOMA

It is the most common neoplasm seen in HIV infected patients. The cutaneous lesion begins as a red macule that enlarges to become blue, purple and ultimately brown nodular tumefaction. Oral lesions occur on the posterior hard palate. It begins as a flat red macule of variable size and irregular configuration. It is multifocal and involves the whole palate.

HEREDITARY HEMORRHAGIC TELANGIECTATIC

It is a genetically transmitted disease inherited as an autosomal dominant trait. Papules are red or brown rather than purple. It is characterized by multiple, round or oval papules measuring less than 0.5 cm in diameter. There may be hundreds of such purple papules on the vermilion border and mucosal surface of lips as well as tongue and buccal mucosa.

Brown Melanotic Lesions

Labial and Oral Melanotic Macule

It is also called as *'Ephelis'*, *'focal melanosis'* or *'solitary labial Lentigo'*. It represents an increase in synthesis of melanin pigments by basal cell layer melanocytes without increase in the number of melanocytes. It is the most common pigmentation to occur in oral cavity of light skinned individuals.

It is attributed to actinic exposure and therefore occurs on vermilion border of the lower lip. Sometimes it can also

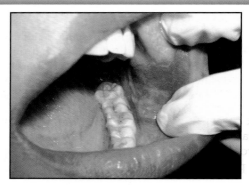

Fig. 10.4: Melanin pigmentation appear as labial melanotic macule

occur on gingiva, palate and buccal mucosa. It present as small, flat macule which may be single or multiple (Fig. 10.4). Brown or brown black pigmentation. Solitary lesion is less than 1 cm in diameter and constant in size. Lesions are oval or irregular in outline. It is an asymptomatic condition.

Excision with Adequate Borders

Melanoplakia

Melanin is produced by dentrite melanocytes in basal cell layer of epidermis and is formed by oxidation of tyrosine, a reaction that is catalyzed by copper containing enzyme *tyrosinase* and mediated by melanocyte stimulating hormone from anterior pituitary.

This term is applied to a flat, localized or widespread, black or brownish discoloration of the oral mucosa due to increased amount of melanin (Fig. 10.5).

It may occur due to smoker's melanosis (Fig. 10.6), racial pigmentation, Peutz-Jegher's syndrome, Addison's disease or hemochromatosis or may result from lead poisoning or cancer chemotherapy.

Dark complexioned people frequently have macular pigmentation of various sizes on their oral mucosa. Color varies from light brown to blue depending on amount of melanin present and depth of lesion.

Nevus and Nevi

It is a congenital or acquired benign tumor of melanocytes. Color range from gray to light brown to blue to black (Fig. 10.7).

Excision with wide border of normal tissue.

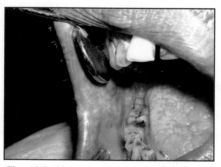

Fig. 10.5: Melanoplakia appear as brownish discoloration of oral mucosa

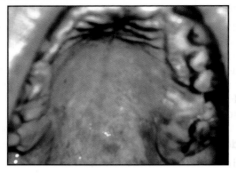

Fig. 10.6: Smoker melanosis seen on hard palate as brownish color

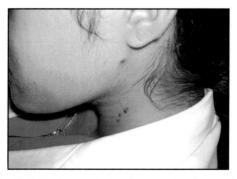

Fig. 10.7: Nevi presented as brown color pigmentation

Melanoma

It is neoplasm of epidermal melanocytes. It appears as macular or nodular and color varies from brown to black to blue with zones of depigmentation. In oral cavity, it appear on anterior labial gingiva and the anterior aspect of the palate. It appears as brown or black plaques with irregular outline (Fig. 10.8).

Excision with wide margins of normal tissue.

Drug Induced Melanosis

The chief drugs implicated are the quinolines, hydroxyquinoline, and amodiaquine antimalarials drugs. Minocycline, used in the treatment of acne, can also produce oral pigmentation. Drug intake for a minimum of 4 months is a must for such pigmentation to occur.

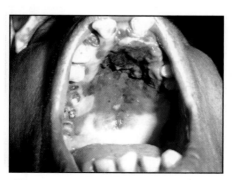

Fig. 10.8: Melanoma presented as brown to black color pigmentation on palate

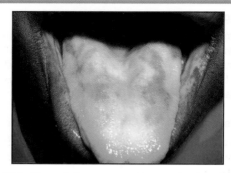

Fig. 10.9: Pigmentation occur on tongue due to quinolines

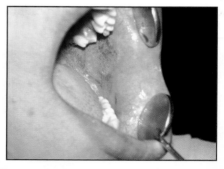

Fig. 10.10: Pigmented lichen planus may occur due to lichenoid reaction

It is gray to blue black (Figs 10.9 and 10.10), large but localized to hard palate or multifocal throughout the mouth.

Physiologic Pigmentation

It is common characteristic of darker races.

Gingiva and tongue are the most common sites. It may exhibit multiple (Fig. 10.11), diffuse, and reticulated brown macules. It can be generalized or localized in uniform or bizarre patterns.

Addison's Disease

It is also called as chronic adrenal insufficiency. It is caused by bilateral adrenocortical destruction after tuberculosis for fungal infection.

Abnormal pigmentation of the skin and mucous membrane. Cheek most common site followed by gingiva, tongue and lips. Bronzing of skin (Fig. 10.12), pigmentation

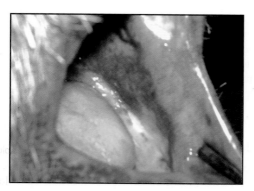

Fig. 10.11: Diffuse type of pigmentation
due to physiological process

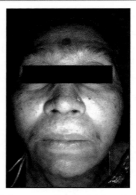

Fig. 10.12: Pigmentation occurring in Addison's disease showing as brown to black color pigmentation

of mucus membrane, feeble heart action, generalized debility, nausea, vomiting, diarrhea, and severe anemia. The color of oral mucosa varies from bluish black to pale brown or deep chocolate spreading over the buccal mucosa from the angle of the mouth or developing on the gingiva, tongue and lips.

It is done by adequate corticosteroid maintenance therapy provided by an average daily dose of 25 to 40 mg cortisone.

Peutz-Jeghers Syndrome

It is also called as *'hereditary intestinal polyposis syndrome'*. It consists of familial generalized intestinal polyposis and pigmented spot on face, oral cavity and sometimes on hand

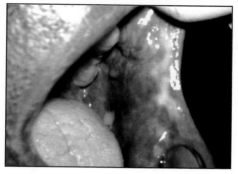

Fig. 10.13: Café-au-lait spot seen in Peutz-Jegher's syndrome

and feet. It is inherited as a simple Mendelian dominant characteristic.

Frequent episodes of abdominal pain and signs of minor obstruction, often terminating in intrussusception. There are *'bluish-black'* macules on skin. The skin pigmentation often fades away in later life. Size is 1-5 cm in diameter. On the face, spot tends to be grouped around eye, nostril and lips. Facial pigmentation tends to fade in later life.

Orally intraorally common on buccal mucosa, gingiva, tongue, hard palate, and tongue in decreasing order. There are multiple melanotic, brownish, macules concentrated around the lip (Fig. 10.13). They are 0.5 cm in diameter.

Surgical intervention is required for intrussusception.

Neurofibromatosis

It is also called as *'von Recklinghausen's disease'*. It is transmitted as autosomal dominant trait. In it, multiple neurofibromas of the skin along with brown spots are seen.

Clinical triad consists of areas of pigmentation, sessile or pedunculated tumors of skin and mucous membrane and tumors of nerves. Tumors are of plexiform variety and thus are soft, smooth, fluctuant, flesh colored and nodular or pedunculated. Multiple cavernous neurofibromas and auxiliary folding can be seen. *Café-au-lait spots*—are cutaneous lesions which are characteristic of the disease.

Orally areas of melanin pigmentation are seen on oral mucosa with lips being the common site of involvement (Fig. 10.14). Jaws can be involved by intrinsic bone formation,

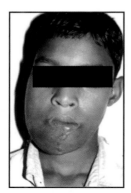

Fig. 10.14: Neurofibromatosis presented with pigmentation on the lip mucosa

presence of extrinsic tumor which involves bone or by tumor which does not actually involve the bone but does influence its growth and its shape.

Radiologically in intrinsic bone tumors, there are actual tumor masses within the bone which appear as central cyst like radiolucency, subperiosteal bone blister and irregular areas of bone destruction. Extrinsic bone tumor produces area of bone destruction or prevents normal development of contour of the bone.

Surgical excision of individual lesion

Albright's Syndrome

A type of fibrous dysplasia involving all the bones in the skeleton accompanied by the lesions of the skin and endocrine disturbances of varying types. Skin lesions are irregularly pigmented melanotic spots described as café-au-lait spots due to their light brown color. It is more common on lips.

BROWN HEME ASSOCIATED LESION
Ecchymoses and Petechiae

They are purpuric submucosal and subcutaneous hemorrhages. Petechiae are minute pinpoint hemorrhages while ecchymosis is larger than 2 cm in diameter.

It occur immediately following traumatic event and erythrocyte extravasation into submucosa. It appears as bright red macule or swelling, if hematoma is formed (Fig. 10.15). After hemoglobin is degraded to hemosiderin, lesion assumes brown color.

Surgery, after detection of disease.

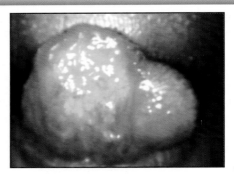

Fig. 10.15: Hematoma seen in tongue as bluish red swelling

Hemochromatosis

It is also called as *'bronze diabetes'*. It is tetrad of liver cirrhosis, diabetes, cardiac failure and bronze skin.

It is caused by increased dietary iron intake and excessive blood transfusions. It is characterized by deposition of excess irons (ferritin and hemosiderin) into the body tissue resulting in fibrosis and functional insufficiency of involved organs. Tanning occurs due to increased melanin production. Blue gray color of skin especially over genitals, face and arms.

Carotenemia

Chronic excessive levels of carotene pigments due to long and continuous consumption of food containing carotene such as carrots, sweet potatoes and egg. An orange to yellow pigmentation of skin and oral mucosa occurs. Color change is more intense on palm, soles and areas of soft palate.

Jaundice

Yellow or green discoloration of the skin and mucous membrane with bile pigments. Oral mucosa presents a yellowish discoloration. Tongue is heavily coated.

EXOGENOUS PIGMENTATION

It is defined as a pigmentation which arises as a result of introduction of metal/drugs into the body via mucous membrane, intestinal tract and skin.

Amalgam Tattoo

It may be condensed in the abraded gingiva during routine amalgam restorative work.

It is described as a flat macule or sometimes slightly raised lesion with margins being well-defined or diffuse in other. Pigmentation is blue black in color (Fig. 10.16). It may gradually increase in size.

Treatment is not necessary. However, if required, excision is done.

Bismuthism

It is cause by medicinal use of bismuth containing preparation.

Vague gastrointestinal tract disturbances, nausea, bloody diarrhea, *'bismuth grippe'* and jaundice. *Bismuth line*

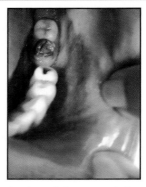

Fig. 10.16: Amalgam tattoo presented as blue black
pigmentation presented as the side of filling

- sometimes in the long bone, white bands of increase density appear in the ends of the diaphyses immediately adjacent to the epiphyseal lines. This is called as 'bismuth line'.

Orally patients often complain of a metallic taste with burning sensation in the oral cavity and annoying gingivostomatitis with symptoms similar to ANUG. Large, extremely painful, shallow ulcerations are seen at times on the cheek mucosa in molar region. Blue black' bismuth line appears to be well demarcated to eye on gingival papillae.

Plumbism

It occurs due to lead poisoning. It is caused by lead in the paints, glazes, cooking vessels, batteries, ointment and containers. 'Moonshine' an illicit alcoholic beverage distilled in car radiators has been shown to cause acute lead poisoning.

Nervous system—Lead has high affinity for cells in central as well as peripheral systems. In acute poisoning, demyelination and axon degeneration occurs. Lead encephalopathy, cerebral palsy, mental retardation, seizures, wrist or foot drop and fatigue can occur.

Gastrointestinal tract—There may be serious gastro-intestinal disturbances like nausea, constipation, vomiting, and colic.

Bone—When incorporated in the bone it can interfere with cellular metabolism and changes the rate of bone resorption and apposition.

Orally there is a metallic taste which is accompanied by excessive salivation and dysphagia. *Burtonian line* - when exposure to lead is very high and oral hygiene is very poor, a line known as 'burtonian line' is seen which is gray black in color and is present along the gingival margin (Fig. 10.17). Lead line is more diffuse than bismuth line. There is bilateral parotid gland hypertrophy.

Lead can be removed from body by using a chelating agent such as calcium edetate (EDTA) or penicillamine.

Argyria

It is also called as *'argyrosis'* which occurs due to chronic exposure to silver compound.

It is cause by local and systemic absorption of silver compounds. It may result from the use of silver containing nasal drops or sprays or silver-arsphenamine injection used to treat syphilis.

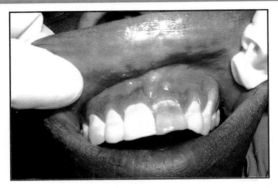

Fig. 10.17: Gray-black line seen in plumbism on the gingiva

The exposed body surfaces including the nail beds are deeply discolored. Skin is slate gray, violet or cyanotic and in marked cases, there is even suggestion of metallic luster.

Orally pigmentation is distributed diffusely throughout the gingival and mucosal tissue.

Source of contact should be eliminated.

LOCALIZED PIGMENTATION

Chlorhexidine Stains

Prolonged use of this mouth wash imparts a yellowish-brown to brown color to the tissues of the oral cavity. Appears in the cervical and interproximal regions of the teeth.

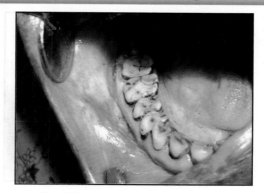

Fig. 10.18: Tobacco stains also occurring on gingiva of the patient

Hairy Tongue

It involves dorsum in middle and posterior thirds of the tongue. Pigmented colonization of bacteria, tobacco and foods. The color of pigmentation is green to brown to black.

Tobacco Stains

It is tenacious dark brown or black surface deposits with brown discoloration of the tooth substances (Fig. 10.18). Staining results from coal tar.

TETRACYCLINE ADMINISTRATION

Discoloration of either deciduous or permanent teeth may occur as a result of prophylactic or therapeutic regimen instituted for pregnant females or infants. May cause

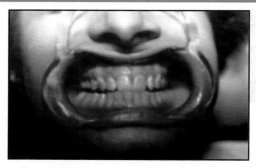

Fig. 10.19: Tetracycline staining of gray-brown color seen in the teeth

discoloration during formation period, tetracycline react with calcium to form calcium orthophosphate complex. It also causes enamel hypoplasia which may be seen in primary as well as in permanent teeth. It is deposited during mineralization and can be demonstrated as golden fluorescence in ultraviolet light, which is more intense in dentin than enamel. Bands are more intense toward DEJ (Fig. 10.19). It shows yellow to brown discoloration of teeth. The location coincides with the part of tooth developing at the time of administration of tetra-cycline.

It is usually seen with different color in different form of tetracycline.

- *Chlortetracycline* - gray-brown
- *Oxytetracycline* – yellow
- *Demeclocycline* – yellow
- *Doxycycline* – there is no changes in teeth color.

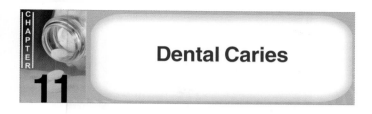

Dental Caries

Interproximal Caries

It takes 3 to 4 years to manifest clinically as loss of enamel transparency resulting in opaque chalky region (white spot). In some cases it appears as a yellow or brown pigmented area but it is usually well demarcated. Spots are generally located on the outer surface of enamel between contact point and height of free gingival margin.

The early white chalky spot becomes slightly roughened owing to superficial decalcification of the enamel (Fig. 11.1). As the caries penetrates the enamel, the enamel surrounding the lesion assumes bluish white appearance which is usually apparent as laterally spreading caries at the dentinoenamel junction. Caries do not initiate below free gingival margin. It is common for proximal caries to extend both buccally and lingually (Fig. 11.2).

Radiographic detection of carious lesion on proximal surfaces of teeth depends on loss of enough material to result in detectable changes in radiographic density. As the proximal surfaces of posterior teeth are often broad, the loss of small amounts of mineral is difficult to diagnose on

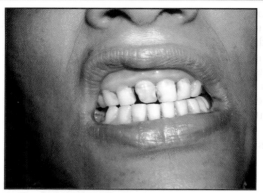

Fig. 11.1: Interproximal caries seen on right and left central incisor area

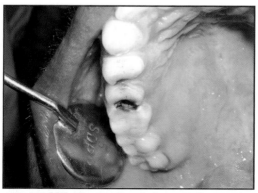

Fig. 11.2: Proximal carious lesion seen in second molar and first molar in upper area

radiograph. Interproximal carious lesions of enamel are triangular in shape and decrease in volume as they progress towards dentinoenamel junction (Fig. 11.3). As the carious lesion approaches the DEJ not only does it become smaller but it is superimposed with more and more sound enamel which attenuates the X-ray and tends to obscure the demineralized lesion in proportion to its depth. 20 to 30 percent of demineralization is required for detection of lesion. Radiologically proximal caries is divided into four groups:

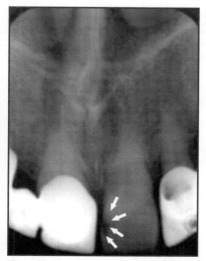

Fig. 11.3: Interproximal caries lesion at the medial side of the maxillary left central incisor tooth (*Courtesy:* Fusan Yasser)

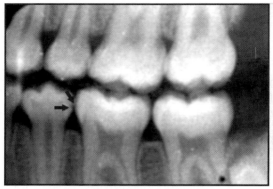

Fig. 11.4: An incipient carious lesion just involving half of the enamel at the distal interproximal area of mandibular second premolar which is not seen clinically

Incipient Caries

Radiographically this caries susceptible zone has vertical dimension of 1.0 to 1.5 mm. There is loss of normal homogeneity of the enamel shadow. Radiologically it appears as a radiolucent notch on the outer surface of teeth (Fig. 11.4).

Moderate Caries

Interproximal incipient lesion that develops and involves more than outer half of enamel but that do not radiographically extends into DEJ may be called moderate lesion (Fig. 11.5). Once the dentin is involved the margins of

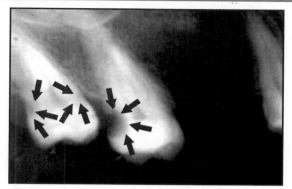

Fig. 11.5: Moderate carious lesion in the maxillary second and third molar tooth

the radiolucent areas tapers off gradually into the adjacent tooth substance.

Advanced Caries

These are lesions that have invaded DEJ. Classically there is more penetration through enamel. Configuration is usually triangular. It may be diffuse or combination of triangular and diffuse. Spreading of demineralization process at DEJ, undermining the enamel and subsequently extending into dentin which forms second irregular radiolucent image in dentin with base at DEJ and apex directed towards pulp.

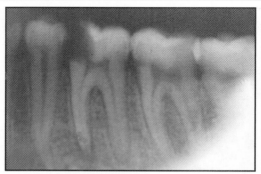

Fig. 11.6: Severe interproximal caries involving mesial surface of mandibular first molar

Severe Caries

When carious lesion is seen radiographically to have penetrated through more than half of dentin and is approaching the pulp chamber it is categorized as severe (Fig. 11.6). It may or may not appear to involve pulp. Force of mastication will cause the undermined enamel to collapse leaving very large cavity or hole in the tooth.

Cervical, Buccal, Lingual or Palatal Caries

It usually extends from the area opposite the gingival crest occlusally to the convexity of the tooth surface. It extends laterally towards the proximal surfaces and on occasion extends beneath the free margin of the gingiva. It usually occurs in cervical area and the typical cervical lesion is a

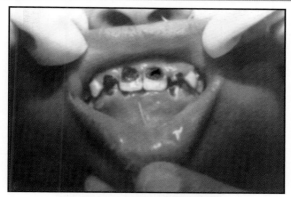

Fig. 11.7: Gross labial caries seen in upper anterior region

crescent shaped cavity beginning as slightly roughened chalky area which gradually becomes excavated (Fig. 11.7).

Radiologically it is difficult to differentiate between buccal and lingual caries on a radiograph. There is uniform radiopaque circular region representing parallel non-carious enamel rod surrounding the buccal or palatal decay (Fig. 11.8). Occlusal caries will be more extensive than lingual and buccal caries and its outline will not be as well-defined.

Pit and Fissure Caries

It is also called as *'occlusal caries'*. It is primary type and develops in the occlusal surface of molars and premolars. Deep narrow pits and fissures favor the retention of food

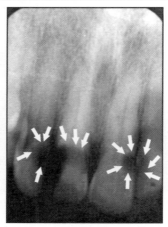

Fig. 11.8: Cole carious lesions in the maxillary anterior teeth

debris and microorganisms and caries may result due to fermentation of this food and the formation of acids.

It usually occurs in pits and fissures with high steep walls and narrow bases. It appears brown or black (Fig. 11.9) and will feel slightly soft and catch a fine explorer point. Thus there may be large carious lesion with only a tiny point of opening.

Radiologically

Incipient Lesion

Radiograph is not effective for the detection of an occlusal caries unless it reaches the dentin. The only change at the

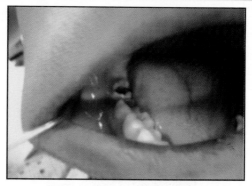

Fig. 11.9: Pit and fissure caries presented as destruction
of occlusal surface in lower right third molar

occlusal surface produced by early lesion is fine gray
shadow just under the DEJ (Fig. 11.10). Carious lesion
generally starts at the side of fissure wall rather than its
base. The lesion tends to penetrate nearly perpendicular to
DEJ.

Moderate Lesion

There is broad based thin radiolucent zone in the dentin
with little or no changes in enamel (Fig. 11.11). There is
band of increased opacity between carious lesion and pulp
chamber.

Severe Lesion

Large hole or cavity in the crown of the teeth (Fig. 11.12).
Masticatory stress causes collapse of enamel.

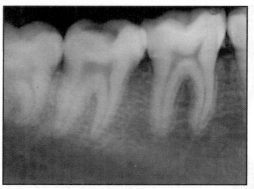

Fig. 11.10: Incipient occlusal caries seen on second molar which is not extended into the dentin

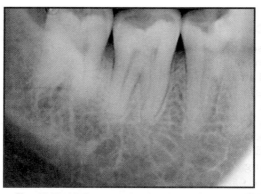

Fig. 11.11: Moderate occlusal caries in first molar which extend into the dentin

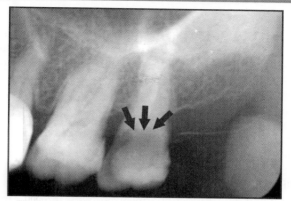

Fig. 11.12: Profound carious lesion in the maxillary left second molar with root canal treatment (missing restoration)

Root Caries

It is also called as *'cemental caries'* and involves both dentin and cementum. Freshly exposed root are more vulnerable to an acid attack because of higher porosity and smaller crystal.

It is usually found in mandibular molar and premolar region. Tooth surface involved in decreasing order of frequency are buccal, lingual, interproximal. Gingival recession is associated with root surface caries.

Radiologically the carious process is best described as scooping out which result in radiographic appearance usually described as ill-defined saucer like crater. If peripheral surface area is small, the appearance of carious lesion will be notched rather than saucer like.

Recurrent Caries

Dental caries that occurs immediately adjacent to the restoration is referred to as recurrent caries. It may be caused by inadequate extension of restoration and without complete excavation of original carious lesion.

Sixteen percent of restored teeth have recurrent caries. Restoration will show poor margins which permitted leakage and the entrance of both bacteria and substrate.

Radiologically teeth have areas of increased radio-lucency along the margins of the restoration (Fig. 11.13).

Rampant Caries

It is defined as a suddenly appearing, widespread, rapidly burrowing type of caries, resulting in early involvement of

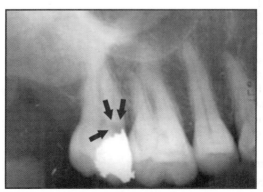

Fig. 11.13: Secondary caries lesion under an amalgam restoration in the maxillary second molar tooth

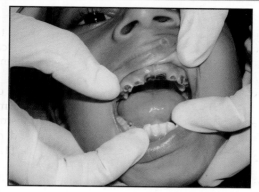

Fig. 11.14: Rampant caries total destruction of tooth surface

the pulp and affecting those teeth usually regarded as immune to ordinary decay. Some believe that the term rampant caries should be applied to those carious lesions with 10 or more new lesions per year.

It usually occurs in children with poor dietary habits. It demonstrates extensive interproximal and smooth surface caries (Fig. 11.14). Rampant caries can occur suddenly in teeth that were for many years relatively immune to decay.

Radiographically demonstrate severe advanced carious lesions especially of mandibular anterior teeth.

Arrested Caries (Fig. 11.15)

It has been described as caries which becomes static or stationary and does not show any tendency for further progression.

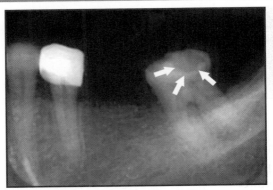

Fig. 11.15: Arrested caries in the left mandibular second molar

Both deciduous and permanent dentitions are affected by this condition. It occurs exclusively in caries of occlusal surfaces. It is characterized by large open cavities in which there is lack of food retention and in which the superficially softened and decalcified dentin is gradually burnished and has taken a brown-stained polished appearance and is hard. This has been referred to as 'eburnation of dentin'. In some cases there is brown stained area at or just below the contact of the affected tooth.

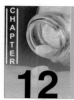

Regressive Changes of Teeth

ATTRITION

It is the physiologic wearing away of teeth because of tooth to tooth contact, as in mastication. It plays an important physiological role as it helps to maintain an advantageous crown-root ratio and gains intercoronal space of 1 cm, which facilitates third molar eruption.

It can be *physiological attrition or pathological attrition. Pathological is caused by abnormal occlusion, abnormal chewing habits,* in certain occupations, workers are exposed to an atmosphere of abrasive dust and cannot avoid it getting into mouth.

The first clinical manifestation of attrition is the appearance of small polished facet on a cusp tip or ridge and slight flattening of an incisal edge.

Physiological Attrition

Physiological attrition beings with wearing of the incisal edge of an incisor, which is followed by the palatal cusp of maxillary molars and buccal cusp of mandibular molars (Fig. 12.1). It commences at the time of contact or occlusion.

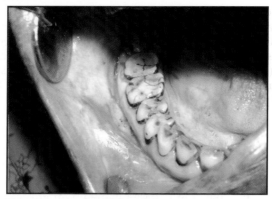

Fig. 12.1: Severe pathological attrition seen in posterior region due to tobacco chewing habit

Physiological tooth surface loss results in a reduction, in both vertical tooth height and horizontal tooth width. When the dentin gets exposed it generally becomes discolored, i.e. brown in color. There is gradual reduction in cusp height and consequent flattening of occlusal inclined plane (Fig. 12.1).

Pathological Attrition

If pathologically vertical dimension of tooth has reduced then, there is the possibility of compensatory growth (dentoalveolar compensation) to some degree. If attrition affecting the occlusal surfaces of teeth has occurred, then reduction in occlusal face height (vertical dimension of occlusion) and increase in the freeway space could be anticipated.

Radiologically smooth wearing of incisal and occlusal surfaces of involved teeth is evident by shortened crown image (Fig. 12.2). Sclerosis of pulp chamber and canals is seen due to deposition of secondary dentin which narrows the pulp canals.

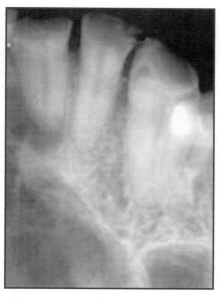

Fig. 12.2: Loss of enamel structure in the incisal third

ABRASION

It is the pathological wearing away of tooth substance through abnormal mechanical process.

It is caused by use of *abrasive dentifrices*, horizontal tooth brushing, habitual opening of bobby pins, *Holding nails* or *pins* between teeth, e.g. in carpenters, shoemakers or tailors. *Improper use* of dental floss and tooth picks.

It can be tooth *brush abrasion, habitual abrasion, occupational abrasion, ritual abrasion* (seen in Africa).

Tooth brush injury—It usually occurs on exposed surfaces of roots of teeth. It occurs due to back and forth movement of brush with heavy pressure causing bristles to assume wedge shaped arrangement between crown and gingiva (Fig. 12.3). In horizontal brushing there is usually a

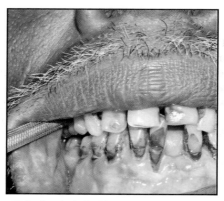

Fig. 12.3: Cervical abrasion seen due to faulty tooth brushing habit. It appear as semicircular shape

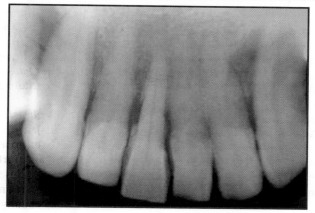

Fig. 12.4: Cervical abrasion seen as semicircular radiolucency in the cervical area

'*V*' shaped or '*wedge*' shaped ditch on the root at cemento-enamel junction. Patient develops sensitivity as dentin becomes exposed. Cervical lesions caused purely by abrasion have sharply defined margins and a smooth, hard surface. Exposed dentin appears highly polished.

Dental floss or tooth prick injury - cervical portion of proximal surfaces, just above the gingival margin, is affected. Grooves on distal surface are deeper than on mesial surface.

Radiologically radiolucent defect at the cervical level of teeth (Fig. 12.4). Well-defined semilunar shape, with borders of increasing density. Pulp chamber may be partially or fully sclerosed in severely affected teeth.

EROSION

It is the loss of tooth substance by chemical process that does not involve known bacterial action. Dissolution of mineralized tooth structure occurs upon contact with acids.

It can be *intrinsic* – erosion that occur due to intrinsic cause, e.g. gastroesophageal reflux, vomiting and *extrinsic* –erosion occurring from extrinsic sources, e.g. acidic beverages, citrus fruits.

It is usually a smooth lesion which exhibits no chalkiness. Loss of tooth substance is manifested by shallow, broad, smooth, highly polished and scooped out depression on enamel surface adjacent to cementoenamel junction. There may be pink spot on tooth which is attributable to the reduced thickness of enamel and dentin making the pink hue of pulp visible. When erosion affects the palatal surfaces of upper maxillary teeth, there is often a central area of exposed dentine surrounded by a border of unaffected enamel.

Radiologically it appears as radiolucent defect in the crown margins may be well-defined or diffuse.

ABFRACTION

It is also called as *'stress lesion'* It has been suggested that the stress lesion or abfraction is a consequence of eccentric forces on the natural dentition. The theory propounds tooth fatigue, flexure and deformation via biomechanical loading of the tooth structure, primarily at the cervical region. Cusp flexure causes stress at the cervical fulcrum and results in loss of the overlying tooth structure.

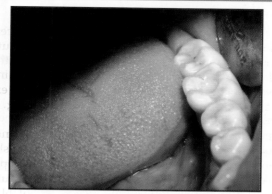

Fig. 12.5: Occlusal abfraction seen as circular invagination in first molar area

It appears as deep, narrow V-shaped notch. The lesion is typically wedge shaped with sharp line angles, but occlusal abfraction may present as circular invaginations (Fig. 12.5). The magnitude of tooth tissue loss depends on the size, duration, direction, frequency and location of the forces.

RESORPTION OF TEETH

It is chronic progressive damage or loss of tooth structure due to the action of cells called odontoclasts. It can be *physiological* as in case of root resorption of deciduous teeth or *pathological,* which occurs in permanent teeth. Pathological resorption may be *external* or *internal.*

EXTERNAL RESORPTION

It is lytic process occurring in the cementum or cementum and dentin of the roots of teeth.

It is caused by resorption associated with periapical infection, reimplanted teeth, tumors and cysts, excessive mechanical and occlusal forces, impacted teeth, overhanged root canal filling material.

The affected tooth is usually asymptomatic. The most frequent site for external resorption is upper incisors, upper and lower bicuspids. When the root is completely resorbed, the tooth may become mobile. If root resorption is followed by ankylosis then the tooth is immobile, in infraocclusion and with high percussion sound.

Radiologically when the lesion begins at the apex, it causes smooth resorption of the root surface. The conical end is removed and replaced by more or less blunt or usually square apex. Bone and lamina dura show normal appearance. It appears as concave and ragged area on the root surface (Fig. 12.6). If it involves lateral aspect of the tooth, the lesion will be irregular. In external internal resorption it appears as eccentrically shaped notch with areas of resorption which are uneven and appears like trabeculae.

INTERNAL RESORPTION

It is a condition starting in the pulp, in which the pulp chamber or the root canals or both, of the tooth expand by resorption of the surrounding dentin.

It is caused by idiopathic, inflammatory hyperplasia of the pulp, direct and indirect pulp capping, pulpotomy, enamel invagination, acute trauma to teeth and pulp polyp.

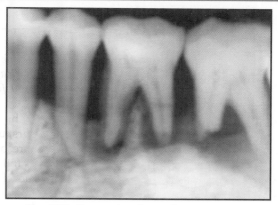

Fig. 12.6: Concaved and ragged areas are seen
on the lateral aspect of the tooth root

Appearance of pink hued area on the crown of tooth,
which represents hyperplastic pulp tissue fitting the
resorbed area and showing through the remaining overlying
tooth substance. It is asymptomatic.

The roots of teeth with internal resorption may manifest
a reddish area, called the 'pink spot'. This reddish area
represents granulation tissue showing through the resorbed
area of crown (Fig. 12.7). When the lesion is located in the
crown of teeth, it may expand to such an extent that the
crown shows dark shadow due to necrosis of the pulp tissue.

Radiologically lesion is radiolucent, round, oval or
elongated within the root with widening of pulp chamber
or canals (Fig. 12.8). The destruction may be symmetrically

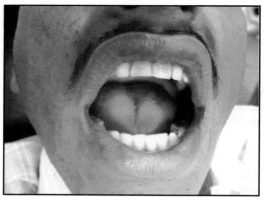

Fig. 12.7: Pink tooth appear due to internal resorption of tooth

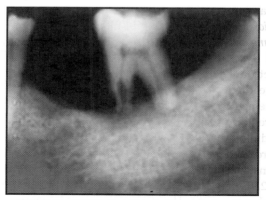

Fig. 12.8: Internal resorption in the root of molar

situated around the original canal or it may be eccentric, so that it is situated entirely on one side of the root. The tooth substance which is destroyed in the root may assume any shape; rounded oval, inverted, pear or irregular. The margins of enlarged chamber are sharp and clearly defined.

Extirpation of pulp with routine endodontic treatment or retrograde filling stops the internal resorption process. Extraction of the tooth, if perforation occurs.

HYPERCEMENTOSIS

It is also called as *'cementum hyperplasia'* or *'exostosis of root'*. It is characterized by deposition of excessive amount of cementum on the root surface. New tissue formation is in direct contact with the cementum of roots of teeth.

It can be *localized* or *generalized*. *It is caused by accelerated elongation of a tooth, inflammation of the root, tooth repair; osteitis deformans or Paget's disease of bone,* hyperpituitarism, cleido-cranial dysostosis can also cause hypercementosis.

Teeth are vital and not sensitive to percussion. There may be difficulty in extraction of teeth. In some cases hypercementosis is so extensive that it causes fusion of two or more adjacent teeth.

Radiologically there is thickening and apparent blunting of root with rounding of apex. Apex appears bulbous in some instances, after symmetrical distribution of cementum (Fig. 12.9). Lamina dura will follow the outline of teeth in normal periodontal ligament space. If cementum is

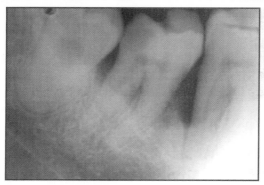

Fig. 12.9: Hypercementosis in association with third molar (*Courtesy:* Dr Ashok L Professor and Head, Oral Medicine and Radiology, Bapuji Dental College and Hospital, Davanagere, India)

distributed eccentrically there is a localized protuberance. There is excessive build of cementum around all or parts of teeth.

Treatment of the primary cause should be done.

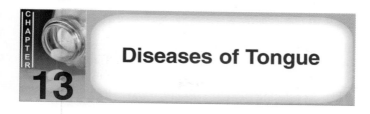

CHAPTER 13

Diseases of Tongue

CONGENITAL AND DEVELOPMENTAL DISORDERS

Aglossia and Microglossia

Aglossia: It is the complete absent of tongue at birth.

Microglossia: It is the presence of small rudimentary tongue.

It usually occurs in syndromes such as hypoglossia-hypodactylia syndrome, Pierre-Robin syndrome. It is also associated with cleft lip and palate.

Patient encounters difficulty in eating and speaking. Patient may have high arched palate and a narrow constricted mandible. It is usually associated with other oral or generalized malformations.

Macroglossia

Macroglossia is tongue enlargement, which leads to functional and cosmetic problems. Although this is a relatively uncommon disorder, it may cause significant morbidity. Normal speech and swallowing reflexes require normal tongue anatomy and function.

It can be *congenital, acquired, hypertrophic, inflam-matory, neoplastic, relative macroglossia* (normal sized tongue appears abnormally large, if it is particularly enclosed within a small oral cavity) and apparent macroglossia (tongue appears large due to poor muscular control of the tongue, although there is no increase in the bulk of tongue tissue).

It is caused by hemangioma, lymphangioma, lingual thyroid, tuberculosis, actinomycosis, dental infection, syphilitic gumma, Riga disease, ranula and sublingual calculus, dental irritation, hematoma, postoperative edema, neoplastic, myxedema, amylodosis, lipoid proteinosis, chronic steroid therapy, acromegaly and muscular hypertrophy (Fig. 13.1).

There is tongue protrusion, which exposes the tongue to trauma. This exposure also leads to mucosal drying and recurrent upper respiratory tract infections. Other symptoms

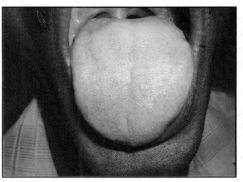

Fig. 13.1: Macroglossia occur due to muscular hypertrophy

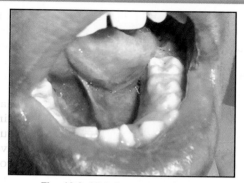

Fig. 13.2: High frenum attachment
seen in the case of tongue

include swallowing difficulties, airway obstruction, drooling and failure to thrive. It may produce displacement of teeth and malocclusion, due to the strength of muscles involved and pressure exerted by the tongue on teeth. Crenation or scalloping of the lateral borders of the tongue; the tips of scalloping fit into the interproximal spaces between the teeth.

Ankyloglossia

It is also called as 'tongue-tie'. It is a condition in which the lingual frenulum is either too short or anteriorly placed (Figs 13.2 and 13.3) limiting the mobility of the tongue.

It can be complete and partial.

It may limit the movement of the tongue. In extreme cases of ankyloglossia, nursing and feeding problems can occur.

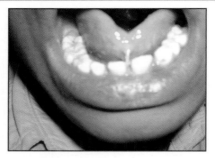

Fig. 13.3: Tongue tie restricting tongue movement

It was felt that tongue-tie was associated with speech abnormalities, especially lisping and inability to pronounce certain sounds and words viz t, d, n, l, as, ta, te, time, etc. Patients have midline mandibular diastema and inability to clean the teeth and lick the lips with tongue.

Cleft Tongue

It is also called as *'bifid tongue'*. It is the condition in which there is cleavage of the tongue due to lack of fusion of the lateral halves. Partially cleft tongue is manifested as deep grooves in the midline of dorsal surface (Fig. 13.4). Food debris and microorganisms may collect in the base of cleft and cause irritation.

Lingual Varices

A varix is a dilated, tortuous vessel, most commonly a vein, which is subjected to increased hydrostatic pressure and is

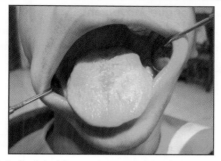

Fig. 13.4: Partial cleft tongue presented as groove in midline

poorly supported by the surrounding tissues. Varices involving the lingual veins are relatively common, appearing as red or purple shotlike clusters of vessels on the ventral surface and lateral borders of the tongue (Fig. 13.5) as well as in the floor of the mouth.

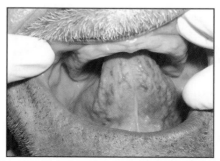

Fig. 13.5: Varices seen as dilated tortuous vessels

Variations in Tongue Movement

Ability to curl up the lateral borders of the tongue into a tube is noted. It is inherited as an autosomal dominant trait.

Trefoil tongue—Clover leaf pattern.

Gorlin sign—Extensibility of the tongue, both, forward to touch the tip of nose and backwards into the pharynx.

Lingual Cyst

It is movable and compressible (Fig. 13.6). It arises as a result of epithelial entrapment during fissural closure of the lateral lingual processes.

Surgical excision is recommended.

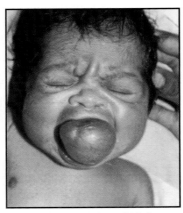

Fig. 13.6: Lingual cyst in infant which is compressible

LOCAL TONGUE DISORDERS

Fissured Tongue

It is also called as 'scrotal tongue', 'plicated tongue' and 'lingua dissecta'.

A tongue with or without a central fissure shows parallel fissures lateral to the midline or fissures at right angle to the long axis of the tongue (Fig. 13.7). A tongue being characterized by furrows, one extending anteroposteriorly and others laterally over the entire anterior surface (Fig. 13.8).

Well marked fissuring increases with age, as does the number, width and depth of the fissures in affected individuals. It is usually painless, except in some occasional

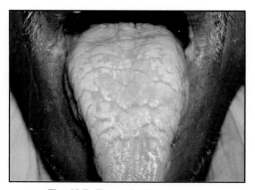

Fig. 13.7: Fissured tongue seen as multiple groove in the tongue

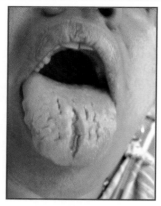

Fig. 13.8: Fissured tongue presented as deep
multiple groove in the anterior surface of tongue

cases in which food debris tends to collect in the groove and
produce irritation. Six different patterns of tongue fissuring
were observed, i.e. plication, central longitudinal fissuring,
double fissures, and transverse fissuring arising from a
central fissure, transverse fissuring with a central fissure
and lateral longitudinal fissuring.

Median Rhomboid Glossitis

It is also called as 'central papillary atrophy of tongue'. It is
a developmental defect resulting from an incomplete desent
of tuberculum impar and entrapment of a portion between
fusing lateral halves of the tongue.

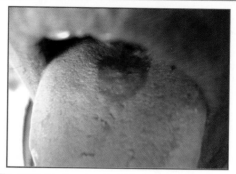

Fig. 13.9: Median rhomboidal glossitis presented as
devoid papillae in the tubercular impair area

It is a benign lesion of the tongue, characterized by
rhomboid or oval shaped changes of the tongue mucosa in
the midline, just anterior to the foramen cecum (Fig. 13.9).

It appears as an ovoid, diamond or rhomboidal shaped
reddish patch or plaque on the dorsal surface of the tongue,
immediately anterior to the circumvallate papillae. In some
cases flat or slightly raised area stands out from rest of the
tongue because it has no filiform papillae. The surface is
dusky red and completely devoid of filiform papillae and
usually smooth. Rest of the tongue may be coated or matted.

Benign Migratory Glossitis

It is also called as *'geographic tongue'*, *'wandering rash'*, 'and
glossitis areata exfoliativa 'and *'erythema migrans'*.

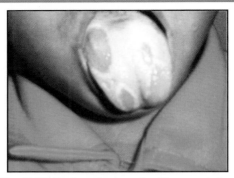

Fig. 13.10: Benign migratory glossitis presented as erythematous area in a child patient

It refers to irregularly shaped reddish areas of depapillation and thinning of dorsal tongue epithelium that is surrounded by a narrow zone of regenerating papillae that are whiter than the surrounding tongue surface (Fig. 13.10).

It is asymptomatic, but the patient may complain of burning sensation that is made worse by spicy or citrous food. Initially appears as a small erythematous, non-indurated, atrophic lesion, bordered by a slightly elevated distinct rim that varies from gray to white to light yellow. Loss of filiform papillae produces pink to red smooth shiny surface except the residual fungiform papillae.

Multiple areas of desquamation of filiform papillae, in an irregular circinate fashion are seen (Fig. 13.11). Fungiform papillae persist in the desquamated areas as small elevated red rods. Area of desquamation remains for a short time in

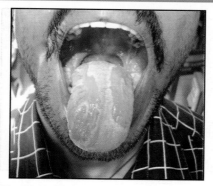

Fig. 13.11: Typical case of migratory glossitis showing multiple area of desquamation

one location and then heals and appears in another location thus giving rise to the term 'migration'.

Topical local anesthetic agents like lidocaine, dyclonine hydrochloride or diphenhydramine can be given. Bland diet, elimination of irritants and psychological reassurance is useful. Topical corticosteroids and topical application of salicylic acid and tretinoin (retinoic acid or vitamin A) for external use.

Hairy Tongue

It is also called as 'lingua villosa'. It designates an overgrowth of the filiform papillae on the dorsum of the tongue, giving the tongue a superficial resemblance as that of hairiness.

It is caused by increase in the rate of formation of keratin, *Candida albicans*, anemia, gastric upset, drugs like sodium perborate, sodium peroxide and antibiotics like penicillin and Aureomycin, extensive X-ray radiation around head and neck.

Papillae which are of considerable length will occasionally brush the palate and may produce gagging. There is hypertrophy of filiform papillae. The papillae may reach a length of 2 cm. The papillae are elongated, sometimes markedly so and have the appearance of hair. The hyperplastic papillae then become pigmented by the colonization of chromogenic bacteria, which can impart a variety of colors ranging from green to brown to black. This gives it a coated or hairy appearance and retains debris and pigments from substances such as food, tobacco, smoke and candy. Color may be varied from yellowish white (Fig. 13.12) to brown or even black depending upon their staining by extrinsic factors such as tobacco, certain foods, medicines or chromogenic organisms of the oral cavity.

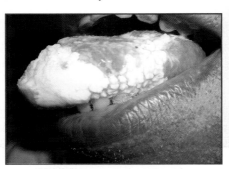

Fig. 13.12: Hairy tongue appearance seen in debilitated patient

The topical application of podophyllum in acetone and alcohol suspension seems to be quite effective. Application of topical keratolytic agents.

Crenated Tongue

The term is applied to a condition in which indentations of teeth are observed at the lateral margins of the tongue.

It may occur due to abnormal tongue pressure habits and tongue thrusting habits. Any enlargement of the tongue may cause indentations on the teeth.

Often, impression of teeth is seen on the tongue (Fig. 13.13). It is usually an asymptomatic and harmless condition.

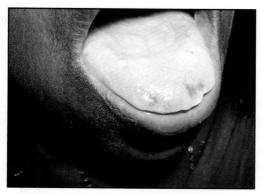

Fig. 13.13: Crenated tongue showing indentation at the anterior surface

Leukokeratosis Nicotina Glossi

It is also called as 'smoker's tongue'. It is homogenous, like leukoplakia with evenly distributed, pinpoint, hemispherical depressions, showing a so called golf ball appearance.

As a result of heavy smoking, there is loss of papillae. No other clinical features are found in these patients.

DEPAPILLATION OF THE TONGUE

Local Disease

Eosinophilic Granuloma

It is not related with eosinophilic granuloma of bone. It is also called as 'ulcerated granuloma eosinophilicum diutinum', 'traumatic granuloma' or 'reparative lesion'. It is characterized by a well demarcated proliferative ulceration covered by thick masses of fibrin and detritus. The lesions are ulcerative, not indurated and rather well circumscribed. There is putrid odor.

Traumatic Injuries

The tongue may be repeatedly traumatized, either mechanically or chemically. Associated with jagged teeth, rough margins of restorations and inadvertent contact of tongue with dental medicaments such as phenol and eugenol. Localized area of depapillation are often noted with papillary regeneration around such areas. Severe damage of the tongue may occur during epileptic seizures.

Lesions due to Automutilation

Injuries to the tongue can occur due to self inflicted bites. It usually occurs in mentally handicapped persons.

Allergic Stomatitis

It refers to edematous changes in part or all of the oral and lingual mucosa, due to hypersensitivity reaction. It can occur due to certain drugs like antibiotics, cancer chemotherapeutic agent and anticholinergic agents. It can also occur due to variety of allergens such as monomer of the denture, mouthwashes, chewing gum and lipstick. There is edematous swelling of the tongue. There is depapillation of the tongue (Fig. 13.14).

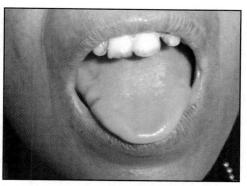

Fig. 13.14: Allergic stomatitis presented as depapillation of the tongue

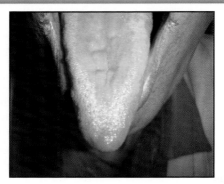

Fig. 13.15: Chronic atropic candidiasis presented at depapillation is in the center

Chronic Candidiasis

Chronic atrophic candidiasis can be present on the dorsum of the tongue (Fig. 13.15). It is difficult to distinguish it from median rhomboidal glossitis. It is diagnosed by scraping and cytological examination.

SYSTEMIC DISEASE

Iron Deficiency Anemia

There are atrophic changes on the dorsum of the tongue. It first appears at the tip and lateral borders with loss of filiform papilla. In extreme cases, the entire dorsum becomes smooth and glazed (Fig. 13.16). The tongue may be very painful and is either pale or fiery red.

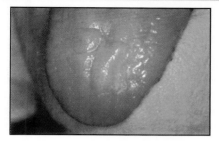

Fig. 13.16: Depapillation of tongue seen in anemia

Pernicious Anemia

The patient suffers from general weakness, burning or itching sensation from the oral mucous membrane with disturbance of taste and occasional dryness of mouth. There may be paresthesia, atrophy of filiform and fungiform papillae (Fig. 13.17). In advanced cases, dorsum of the

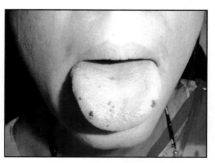

Fig. 13.17: Bleeding from tongue and depapillation seen in patient with pernicious anemia

tongue becomes completely atrophic, smooth and fiery red surface.

Niacin Deficiency

Deficiency of niacin results in a disease called as 'pellagra'. The tongue become fiery red and devoid of papillae. The filiform papillae are most sensitive and disappear first. The fungiform papilla may become enlarged.

Peripheral Vascular Disease

It includes scleroderma and lupus erythematous. Fibrosis of submucosal tissue secondary to the obliteration of small vessels by an autoimmune process is responsible for a scarred, shrunken and atrophic appearance of the tongue in scleroderma. Isolated irregular areas of lingual mucosa, atrophy and ulceration caused by arteritis, are seen in lupus erythematous. In scleroderma the tongue shrinks, losing its mobility and papillary pattern.

Diabetes

Decreased nutritional status of the lingual papillae, as a result of vascular changes affecting sub-papillary dorsal capillary plexus supplying it, causes atrophic glossitis. Central papillary atrophy of the dorsum in which low flat papillae are noticed just anterior to the row of circumvallate papillae, is associated with diabetes.

NEUROLOGICAL DISORDERS

Paralysis

It is also called as 'glossoplegia'. It usually occurs due to unilateral injury of the nucleus in the medulla or the peripheral hypoglossal nerve.

There is paralysis and atrophy of the muscles of one-half of the tongue. The affected tongue deviates towards the paralyzed side when protruded (Figs 13.18 and 13.19). The movement towards the normal side is weak or absent. When the tongue lies on the floor of the mouth, it may deviate or curl slightly toward the healthy side and movements of the tongue towards the back of the mouth on the healthy side, are impaired. In some cases, hypoglossal nerve may be affected bilaterally, causing impairment of the tongue, mobility in lateral direction and atrophy of sides of the tongue.

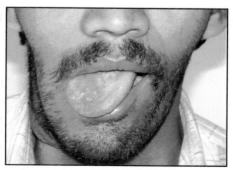

Fig. 13.18: Paralysis of tongue showing movement of tongue on right side

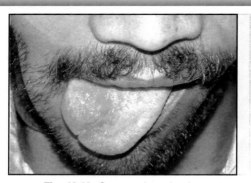

Fig. 13.19: Same patient showing more movement on right side

Squamous Cell Carcinoma

It is the most common oral carcinoma with 60 percent cases arising from the anterior 2/3rd of the tongue and remainder from the base.

It is caused by physical trauma, alcohol, tobacco smoke and candidiasis, syphilis, sepsis, chronic dental trauma, chronic superficial glossitis.

The most common presenting signs of carcinoma of tongue is a painless mass or ulcer, although in most patients the lesion ultimately becomes painful, especially when it becomes secondarily infected. Excessive salivation gradually appears along with the growth. In late stages, saliva becomes blood stained. As the patient is unable to swallow saliva, offensive smell in the mouth occurs due to bacterial stomatitis. There is complained of sore throat and pain in

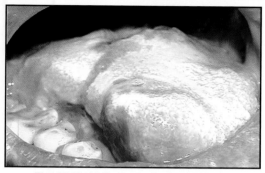

Fig. 13.20: Malignancy of tongue showing ulceration in the body of tongue

case of lesions on posterior border of the tongue. Immobility occurs due to extensive carcinomatous infiltration of the lingual musculature. It becomes worse when floor of mouth is involved and ultimately, it causes difficulty in speech. Hoarseness of voice and dysphagia is present when the carcinoma involves posterior 3rd with involvement of pharynx and larynx. It can be present as ulcerative variety, (Fig. 13.20) warty growth, an indurated (Fig. 13.21) mass and a fissure.

It is managed by surgery, radiotherapy.

MISCELLANEOUS DISORDERS OF THE TONGUE
Pigmentation of Tongue

The tongue may exhibit various patterns of racial melanin pigmentation. Endogenous pigmentation is rarely identi-

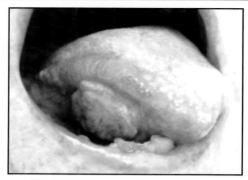

Fig. 13.21: Tongue malignancy showing
indurated ulcer on the lateral border of the tongue

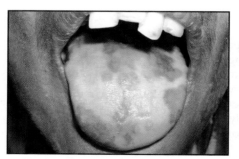

Fig. 13.22: Pigmentation of tongue seen
on the dorsal surface

fiable on the dorsum because of the thickness of the
epithelium, (Fig. 13.22) but jaundice may be apparent under
the thinner ventral mucosa. Exogenous pigmentation of

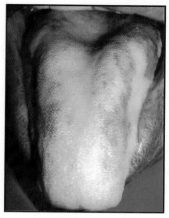

Fig. 13.23: Tongue pigmentation showing bluish discoloration

filiform papillae of the normal (Fig. 13.23) and coated or hairy tongue is very common and result from microbial growth, metabolic products, food debris and dyes from candy, beverages and mouth rinses.

Pigmentation of the tongue has been described by a commonly used anti-chemotherapeutic agent doxorubicin hydrochloride, which also discolor patient's urine, nail beds and skin folds. Extravasation of red cells around lingual varicosities may give patchy, bluish red discoloration. The thin tissue overlying a ranula is said to have a greenish blue appearance.

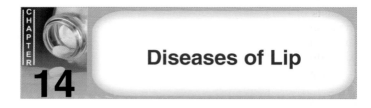

Diseases of Lip

DEVELOPMENTAL DISORDERS

Congenital Lip Pits

It is inherited as autosomal dominant trait. There is notching of lips at an early stage of development with fixation of tissues at the base of the notch. It may occur due to failure of complete union of embryonic sulci of the lip.

Lip pits or fistula is unilateral or bilateral depression. In some cases, sparse mucus secretion may be visible from the base of the pit. Congenital lip pits may occur in association with Van der Woude's syndrome (cleft lip, cleft palate and congenital lip pits)

Surgical excision for cosmetic purpose.

Double Lip

It is an anomaly characterized by a fold of excess tissue on the inner mucosal surface of the lip. It may be congenital or acquired because of trauma to the lip.

When upper lip is tensed double lip resembles 'cupid bow'. It is associated with Ascher's syndrome which consists of double lip, blepharochalasis (it is drooping of the tissue between eyebrow and edge of the upper eyelid so that it hangs loosely over the margin of the lid) and non-toxic thyroid enlargement.

Surgical excision.

Cleft lip and Cleft Palate

It occurs along many planes as a result of fault or defect in the development.

Cleft lip: It is a birth defect that results in a unilateral or bilateral opening in the upper lip between the mouth and the nose. It is also called as harelip. It is wedge shaped defect resulting from failure of two parts of the lip to fuse into a single structure (Fig. 14.1).

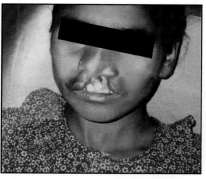

Fig. 14.1: Unilateral cleft lip of the patient which is involving nostril also

Cleft palate: Cleft palate is a birth defect characterized by an opening in the roof of the mouth caused by a lack of tissue development.

It can be unilateral incomplete, unilateral complete, bilateral incomplete and bilateral complete.

Cleft lip: A unilateral cleft involves only one side of the lip; (Fig. 14.2) a bilateral one involves both sides and later gives rise to 'hair lip'. Incomplete cleft extends for varying distances forward to the nostril, but not upto the nostril. The upper part of lip has fused normally. Complete cleft lip extends into nostril and palate is commonly involved. It is often associated with flattening and widening of the nostril of the affected side. Sucking becomes difficult to some extent but not greatly. Defective speech particularly with the labial letters B, F, M, P and V.

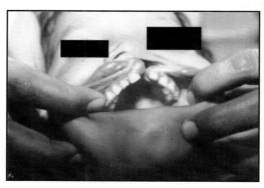

Fig. 14.2: Unilateral cleft lip with involvement of nostril and some portion of palate

Cleft palate: There may be cleft of the hard and soft palate or in some cases, cleft of soft palate alone. Entire premaxillary portion of bone may be missing (Fig. 14.3) and in such instances, the cleft appears to be entirely a midline defect (Fig. 14.4). Cross bite due to medial collapse of pre-maxilla. Eating and drinking is difficult due to regurgitation of food and liquid through the nose. Speech problem is serious and tends to increase due to mental trauma. Cleft of palate may also vary in severity, involving uvula or soft palate or extending all the way through the palate and indirectly to the alveolar ridge on one or both sides. Airway problems may arise in children with cleft palates, especially those with concomitant structural or functional anomalies. Affected patients may develop airway distress from their tongue becoming lodged in the palatal defect. Ear infection and respiratory tract infection.

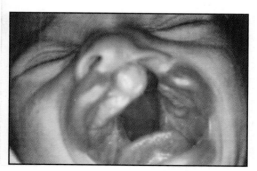

Fig. 14.3: Cleft lip involving palate. Note complete absence of premaxillary portion

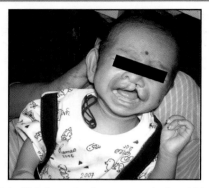

Fig. 14.4: Cleft lip and palate present in the child patient

Radiologically it will determine presence and absence of unerupted teeth. The most common missing teeth are maxillary lateral incisors. There is also presence of supernumerary teeth. Teeth are malformed and poorly positioned. There is also malposition of the teeth in the region of cleft or in the whole maxilla. It will reveal the extent of osseous deformity. There may be complete separation of the premaxilla and maxilla.

It is managed by cheiloplasty, obturator, palatoplasty, bone grafting, orthodontic therapy, cleft rhinoplasty, speech therapy, psychotherapy and feeding plate.

Cheilitis

It is inflammation of lip.

Glandular Cheilitis

It is also called as 'cheilitis glandularis'. It is an uncommon condition in which lower lip becomes enlarged, firm and finally everted.

It is caused by chronic exposure to sun, wind and dust as well as use of tobacco. In several cases, emotional disturbances, as well as familial occurrence, suggesting a hereditary pattern.

It can be simple, superficial suppurative type (Baelz's disease), deep suppurative type (cheilitis glandularis apostematosa, myxadenitis labialis).

Labial salivary glands become enlarged and sometimes nodular. Orifices of secretory ducts are inflamed and dilated appearing as small red macules over the mucosa. Viscid mucous secretion may seep from these openings of everted hypertrophic lips.

Volkmann's cheilitis: It is more severe suppurative form of glandular cheilitis. The lip is considerably and permanently enlarged and is subjected to episodes of pain, tenderness and increased enlargement. The surface is covered by crust and scales beneath (Fig. 14.5) which the salivary duct orifice may be discovered.

It is managed by Vermilionectomy.

Granulomatous Cheilitis

It is also called as 'Miescher's syndrome' or 'cheilitis granulomatosa'. It is a condition of unknown etiology that

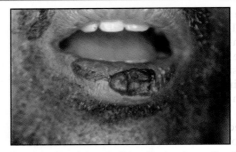

Fig 14.5: Glandular cheilitis affecting lower lip of the patient which is enlarge and scaly

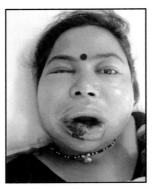

Fig. 14.6: Granulomatous cheilitis showing diffuse edema of and ulceration of lower lip

is not related to chelitis glandularis except by the similarity in the clinical appearance of the two diseases.

There is diffuse swelling of the lips, especially the lower lip (Fig. 14.6). In some cases, an attack is accompanied by fever and mild constitutional symptoms including headache and even visual disturbances. Enlarged lip can create cosmetic problems, difficulty during eating, drinking or speaking. The swelling is usually soft and exhibits no pitting on pressure. Swelling eventually becomes firmer and acquires the consistency of that of hard rubber. It is associated with Melkersson Rosenthal syndrome which consists of fissured tongue and facial paralysis.

Corticosteroid injection and cheiloplasty is done.

Angular Cheilitis

It is also called as 'perleche', 'angular cheilosis'.

It is caused by *Candida albicans*, staphylococci, and streptococci, overclosure of jaws, recurrent trauma from dental flossing, riboflavin, folate and iron deficiency, atopic dermatitis, hypersalivation and Down's syndrome, large tongue and constant dribbling being the contributory factors.

It is usually a roughly triangular area of erythema and edema at one or more, commonly both the angles of mouth (Figs 14.7 and 14.8). Epithelium at the commissures appears wrinkled and somewhat macerated. In time, wrinkling becomes more pronounced to form one or more deep fissures or cracks which appear ulcerated but which do not tend to bleed, although a superficial exudative crust may form. Linear furrow or fissures radiating from the angle of mouth (rhagades) are seen in more severe forms, especially in denture wearers.

Underlying primary cause should be identified and treated. A course of vitamin B and iron supplements is useful

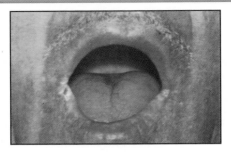

Fig. 14.7: Angular cheilitis present in association
with fissure tongue

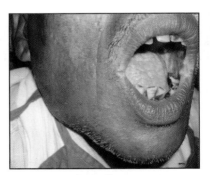

Fig. 14.8: Angular cheilitis present in
association with fissure tongue

in these cases. Fusidic acid ointment, miconazole, gentian
violet application should be done.

Eczematous Cheilitis

The lips are involved secondary to atopic eczema but possibility of contact dermatitis must also be considered. The management of atopic eczema of the lips is with an emollient and topical steroids.

Contact Cheilitis

Contact cheilitis is an inflammatory reaction of the lips provoked by the irritants or sensitizing action of chemical agents in direct contact with them.

It is caused by lipsticks, lipsalves, phenyl salicylates, essential oils such as peppermint, cinnamon, clove, spearmint and bactericidal agents can cause cheilitis. Meury and eugenol may cause cheilitis in the absence of stomatitis.

Lipstick cheilitis is usually confined to the vermilion borders but more often extends beyond that (Fig. 14.9). There

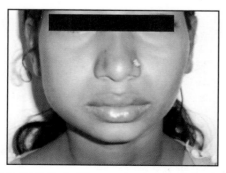

Fig. 14.9: Contact cheilitis occurring in patient due to lipstick

may be persistent irritation and scaling or a more acute reaction with edema and vesiculation

Topical steroids will give symptomatic relief but the offending substance must be traced and avoided.

Actinic Cheilitis

It is also called as 'actinic keratosis' or 'solar cheilosis'.

It is a pre-malignant sq. cell lesion resulting from long term exposure to solar radiation and may be found at the vermilion border of lip as well as other sun exposed surfaces.

In the early stages, there may be redness and edema but later on, the lips become dry and scaly. If scales are removed at this stage, tiny bleeding points are revealed (Fig. 14.10). With the passage of time, these scales become thick and horny with distinct edges. Epithelium becomes palpably

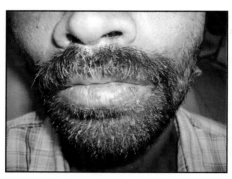

Fig. 14.10: Actinic cheilitis showing some bleeding point on the lip occurring in farmer who work in farm

thickened with small grayish white plaques. At times, vesicle may appear which rupture to form superficial erosions. Secondary infection may occur. Eventually warty nodules may form which tend to vary in size with fluctuation in the degree of edema and inflammation.

It is managed by topical fluorouracil, rapid freezing with CO_2 snow or liquid nitrogen on swab stick, vermilionectomy (lip shaves), laser ablation.

Exfoliative Cheilitis

It is a chronic superficial inflammatory disorder of the vermilion border of lips characterized by persistent scaling. These cases may occur due to repeated lip sucking, chewing or other manipulation of the lips.

It consists of scaling and crusting, more or less confined to the vermilion borders and persisting in varying severity for months or years. The patient complains of irritation or burning and can be observed frequently biting or sucking the lips.

Reassurance and topical steroids are helpful in some cases but in some, psychotherapy or tranquilizers are used.

Drug Induced Cheilitis

Hemorrhagic crusting of the lips is a feature of Stevens-Johnson syndrome which is commonly caused by drugs but, cheilitis can occur as an isolated feature of a drug reaction- either as a result of allergy or a pharmacological effect. The aromatic retinoids, etretinate and isotretinoin cause dryness and cracking of lips in most patients (Fig. 14.11).

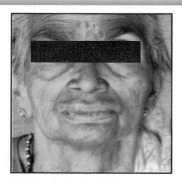

Fig. 14.11: Drug induced cheilitis showing cracking
on both upper and lower lip

Carcinoma of Lip

Squamous cell carcinoma is the commonest malignancy to affect the vermilion zone.

It usually begins on vermilion border of the lip to one side of the midline and it may be covered with a crust due to absence of saliva. It is preceded by actinic cheilitis which is characterized by innocuous looking white plaque on the lip. Patient may complaint of difficulty in speech, difficulty in taking food and inability to close the mouth. There is also pain, bleeding and paresthesia. It often commences as a small area of thickening, induration and ulceration or irregularity of the surface (Fig. 14.12). In some cases it commence as a small warty growth or fissure on the vermilion border of the lip.

Crater like lesion having a velvety red base and rolled indurated borders (Fig. 14.13). As the lesion enlarged it takes

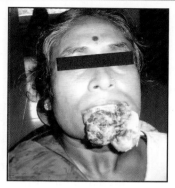

Fig. 14.12: Malignancy involving lip showing ulcerative and extensive growth

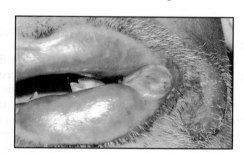

Fig. 14.13: Malignancy involving at the angle of mouth showing induration

papillary or an ulcerative form. In untreated cases there is total destruction of lip and invasion of cheek, the gums and the mandible. It involves submaxillary and submental nodes first and then deep cervical nodes. Spread by direct extension into surrounding structures and by metastasis which is through lymphatic channels.

Surgical excision should be carried out.

MISCELLANEOUS

Chapping of the Lips

It is a reaction to adverse environmental conditions in which keratin of the vermilion zone loose its plasticity, so that lip becomes sore, cracked and scaly. The affected subjects tend to lick the lips or to pick at the scales which may make conditions worse. It is caused by exposure to freezing cold or to hot, dry wind, but acute sunburns can cause very similar changes. Management is by application of petroleum jelly and avoidance of the causative environmental conditions.

Actinic Elastosis

It is also called as 'solar elastosis' or 'senile elastosis'.

It is caused by prolonged exposure to UV light. UV radiation can produce collagen degeneration in the dermis and extent of this effect is dependent upon factors such as the thickness of stratum corneum, melanin pigment, clothing or chemical sunscreens.

Clinical features include leathery appearance, laxity with wrinkling and various pigmentary changes. Clinically, it is manifested in three forms:-

• Cutis rhomdoidalis—thickened skin with furrow giving an appearance of rhomboidal network.
• Dubreuilh's elastoma—diffuse plaque like lesions.
• Nodular elastoidosis—nodular lesion.

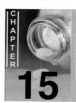

Gingival and Periodontal Diseases

GINGIVAL DISEASES

Fibromatosis Gingiva

It is also called as 'elephantiasis gingivae', 'congenital macrogingivae'. It is a diffuse overgrowth of gingival tissues. It is hereditary. It is autosomal dominant as well as of recessive type.

It is manifested as dense smooth diffuse or nodular overgrowth of gingival tissue of one or both arches (Fig. 15.1) that usually occurs at the time of eruption of teeth. It has a characteristic pebbled surface. In some cases surface has a nodular appearance. Tissue is of normal or pale color. In some cases, it may appear pink. It is often so firm, leathery and dense that it prevents normal eruption of teeth (Fig. 15.2). It is not painful and shows no tendency for hemorrhage. Extent may be such that the crown of fully erupted teeth may be hidden. The dense firm gingival swelling results in varying spacing between the teeth and change in profile and facial appearance.

Surgical removal of excessive tissue with exposure of teeth is necessary.

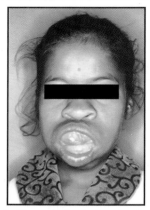

Fig. 15.1: Fibromatosis gingiva showing diffuse overgrowth of gingival tissue

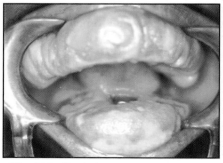

Fig. 15.2: Gingival enlargement preventing the growth of teeth in the jaw

Gingival Inflammation

It is caused by microorganisms (Actinomyces), calculus, food impaction, faulty or irritating restorations or appliances, mouth breathing, tooth malposition, chemical and drug application (phenol, silver nitrates, volatile oils or aspirin). Nutritional disturbances, pregnancy, diabetes mellitus, psychiatric phenomena, hormonal changes.

It may occur in an acute, subacute, or chronic form. It can be localized, generalized, marginal, papillary, diffuse gingivitis.

The earliest symptoms of gingival inflammation are increased gingival fluid production and bleeding from the gingival sulcus on gentle probing. Gingiva become redder when there is an increase in vascularization or when the degree of epithelial keratinization is reduced (Fig. 15.3). The color becomes paler when vascularity is reduced and

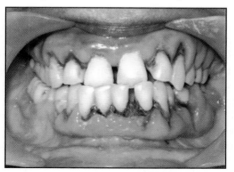

Fig. 15.3: Gingival inflammation seen along with the gingival enlargement both the jaw

keratinization is increased. The color may be sometimes reddish blue or deep blue, if venous stasis has occurred. The color change starts in the interdental papillae, gingival margins and spreads to the attached gingiva. The consistency of gingiva may be spongy that pits on pressure and there may be marked softness of the gingiva. Sometimes in inflammation there may be gingival enlargement and it may lead to changes in the contour of gingiva.

The local irritants should be removed at this stage. Thorough plaque control should be done with scaling and polishing. Use of chlorhexidine, on a short term basis.

Acute Necrotizing Ulcerative Gingivitis

It is an endogenous oral infection that is characterized by necrosis of gingiva. It is also called as 'trench mouth' due to its prevalence in combat trenches. Other synonyms for this are 'Vincent's infection', 'acute ulceromembranous gingivitis', 'fusospirochetal gingivitis' and 'acute ulcerative gingivitis'.

It is caused by fusiform bacilli and spirochetes. In addition to it bacteroides intermedius is also responsible for ANUG. nutritional deficiency, debilitating disease, marked malnutrition, psychosomatic factors.

Onset is sudden with pain, tenderness, profuse salivation and peculiar metallic taste. Spontaneous bleeding from gingival tissue. There is also a loss of sense of taste and diminished pleasure from smoking. The typical fetid odor ultimately develops, which may be extremely unpleasant. Teeth seem slightly to be extruded and are sensitive to pressure or have a woody sensation. They are slightly movable and the patient is unable to eat properly. Gingiva may become superficially stained with brown color. There is blunting of interdental papillae.

A typical lesion consists of necrotic punched out, crater like ulcerations developing most commonly on the interdental papillae and marginal gingiva (Fig. 15.4). Removal of the lesion leaves raw surface. The surface of gingival crater is covered by a gray, pseudomembranous slough, demarcated from the reminder of the gingival mucosa by pronounced linear erythema. Regional lymph nodes are enlarged. There may be a slight elevation of temperature.

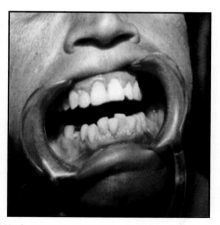

Fig. 15.4: ANUG showing crater like ulceration in interdental papillae

Twice daily rinse with 0.12 percent chlorhexidine are effective. Patients with severe ANUG and lymphadenopathy are treated with antibiotics Penicillin V- 250 or 500 mg, 6 hourly or erythromycin - 250 or 500 mg, 6 hourly with metronidazole 400 mg, 8 hourly, for 7 days are the drugs of choice.

Desquamative Gingivitis

It is a clinical manifestation of several different diseases. It is caused by lichen planus, mucous membrane pemphigoid, bullous pemphigoid or pemphigus, tuberculosis, chronic candidiasis, histoplasmosis, endocrine imbalance, chronic infection and drug reaction, abnormal response to irritation and idiopathic causes, chemical burns.

Gingiva becomes bright red, edematous and desquamation of the surface epithelium of the attached gingiva is also seen (Fig. 15.5). It is usually manifested in three forms

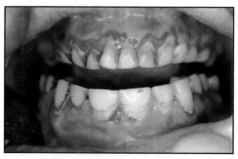

Fig. 15.5: Desquamative gingivitis showing red area and denuded gingiva

mild (diffuse and extends throughout the gingiva), moderate (patchy distribution of bright red and gray areas involving the marginal and attached gingiva, complain of a burning sensation, sensitivity to thermal changes. There is slight pitting on pressure and epithelium is not firmly adherent to the underlying tissues) and severe form (scattered irregularly shaped areas, in which gingiva is denuded and strikingly red in appearance. The overall appearance of gingiva is speckled. A blast of air directed at the gingiva causes elevation of the epithelium and consequent formation of bubbles).

Oxidizing mouth wash (hydrogen peroxide 3 percent diluted to one part peroxide and two parts of warm water) should be use twice daily. Improvement has been noticed with tetracycline therapy. Doxycycline monohydrate 100 gm daily for 4 to 11 weeks.

Topical corticosteroid ointment and creams such as triamcinolone 0.1 percent fluocinolone 0.05 percent is applied and gently rubbed into the gingiva several times daily.

Gingival Abscess

It results from bacteria carried deep into the tissue, when a foreign substance such as a toothbrush bristle, a piece of apple core or a lobster shell fragment is forcefully embedded into the gingiva.

It is localized, painful, rapidly expanding lesion that is usually of sudden onset. In early stages, it appears as a red swelling with a smooth, shiny surface (Fig. 15.6). Within

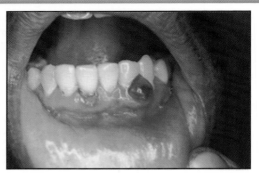

Fig. 15.6: Gingival abscess showing red swelling

24 to 48 hours, the lesion usually becomes fluctuant and pointed with a surface orifice, from which an exudate may be expressed.

After topical anesthetic is applied, the fluctuant area of the lesion is incised with a blade and the incision is gently widened to permit drainage.

Chronic Inflammatory Enlargement

It can be caused by prolonged exposure to dental plaque, food impaction, irritation from clasps or saddle areas of removable prosthesis and nasal obstruction, habits such as mouth breathing can cause gingival enlargement, which is more common in the anterior region.

It originates as a slight ballooning of the interdental papilla or the marginal gingiva. In early stages, it produces a life preserver-like bulge around the involved teeth. It increases in size, until it covers a part of the crown.

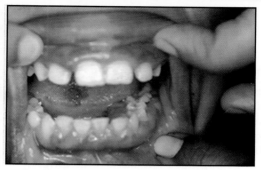

Fig. 15.7: Inflammatory gingival enlargement
showing bluish red enlargement

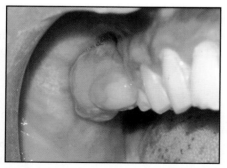

Fig. 15.8: Inflammatory gingival enlargement seen in posterior region

Lesions may be deep red or bluish red (Figs 15.7 and 15.8). They are soft and friable, with a smooth shiny surface and tendency to bleed. It progresses slowly and painlessly, unless complicated by acute infection or trauma. They may undergo spontaneous reduction in size, followed by exacerbation and continued enlargement.

Dilantin Sodium

Dilantin sodium is an anticonvulsant drug, which is used in control of epileptic seizures. Gingival hyperplasia may begin as early as two weeks after dilantin therapy.

The first change noted is a painless bead like enlargement in the size of the gingiva, starting with one or two interdental papillae. The surface of gingiva shows an increase in stippling and finally, a cauliflower, warty or pebbled surface (Fig. 15.9). As the enlargement increases, the gingival tissue becomes lobulated and clefts are seen between each enlarged gingiva (Fig. 15.10). Palpation reveals that the tissue is dense, resilient and insensitive. It

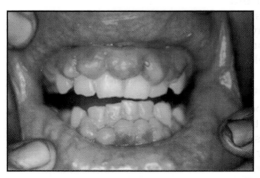

Fig. 15.9: Drug induced enlargement showing bead like enlargement

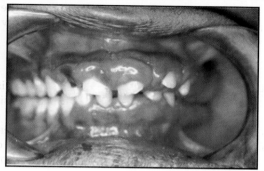

Fig. 15.10: Enlargement occur in the patient
due to use of Dilantin sodium

shows little tendency to bleed. They may interfere with
occlusion. The presence of an enlargement makes plaque
control difficult, resulting in a secondary inflammatory
process that complicates the gingival hyperplasia.

If hyperplasia interferes with function, surgical excision
is recommended. Discontinuing the drug will result in
gradual diminution of the bulk of the gingiva.

Enlargement in Pregnancy

It can be marginal or generalized and may occur as a single
or multiple tumor like masses.

It is an inflammatory reaction to the local irritants. It
usually appears after 3rd month of pregnancy. The lesions
appear as discrete, mushroom like, flattened spherical
masses (Fig. 15.11), that protrude from the gingival margins

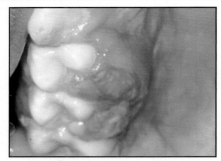

Fig. 15.11: Pregnancy tumor occurring in upper premolar region appearing as mushroom like

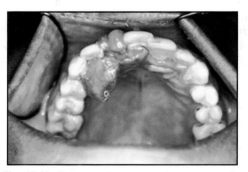

Fig. 15.12: Pregnancy tumor seen in upper anterior region with pedunculated base

or more frequently from the interproximal space and are attached by sessile or pedunculated base (15.12). It tends to expand laterally. The pressure from the tongue and the cheek perpetuates its flattened appearance. It is generally dusky red or magenta; it has a smooth glistening surface that frequently exhibits numerous deep red, pinpoint markings. The consistency varies from semifirm, but may have a varying degree of softness and friability. It is usually painless, unless its size and shape foster the accumulation of debris under its margin or interfere with occlusion, in which cases painful ulceration may occur.

Most gingival enlargement during pregnancy can be prevented by the removal of local irritants and institution of a fastidious oral hygiene.

Enlargement in Puberty

It is usually associated with inflammatory type. It involves mainly the marginal gingivae and interdental gingiva. It is characterized by prominent bulbous interproximal papillae (Fig. 15.13). Sometimes, only facial gingivae are enlarged,

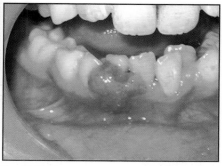

Fig. 15.13: Enlarge gingiva occurring in puberty

as the mechanical action of the tongue prevents heavy accumulation of local irritants on the lingual surface.

After puberty, the enlargement undergoes spontaneous reduction, but does not disappear until local irritants are removed.

Granuloma Pyogenicum

It is a non-specific, tumor-like, conditional enlargement of the gingiva that is considered as an exaggerated conditional response to minor trauma.

It varies from a discrete spherical tumor-like mass with a pedunculated attachment (Fig. 15.14), to a flattened, keloid like enlargement with a broad base. It is bright red or purple color and either friable or firm, depending on its duration.

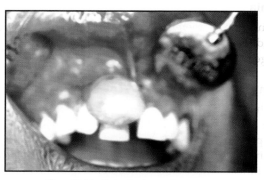

Fig. 15.14: Spherical growth pattern seen in granuloma pyogenicum

In majority of the cases, it presents with surface ulceration and purulent exudation.

Removal of lesion, along with elimination of irritating factors.

SYSTEMIC DISEASES CAUSING ENLARGEMENT AND TUMORS OF GINGIVA

Leukemia

It occurs due to the infiltration of malignant cells into the gingival tissue. The gingiva becomes soft, edematous and swollen. Appearance of gingiva is purplish and glossy. There is also pallor in the surrounding mucosa. Ulceration, pain and severe hemorrhage can also occur.

Anemia

In some case of anemia there may be gingival enlargement. Secondary factor like calculus may be responsible for this enlargement (15.15).

Crohn's Disease

It is characterized by granulomatous superficial ulceration of the intestinal epithelium, with frequent development of multiple fistulae. There is granular and erythematous swelling of gingiva. Other oral feature includes 'cobble stone' appearance of the buccal mucosa with linear hyperplastic folds, diffuse indurated swelling on the lips and multiple ulcerations of the palate.

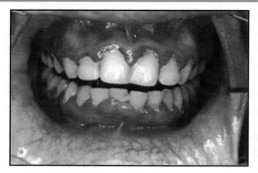

Fig. 15.15: Enlargement of gingiva occurring
in iron deficiency anemia

Vitamin C Deficiency

The gingiva becomes tender, edematous and swollen. There
is ulceration and necrosis of gingiva. It has a spongy
consistency and bleeds frequently. The crest of interdental
papillae appears red or purple.

Orofacial Angiomatosis

Angiomatous proliferation of the gingival blood vessels may
cause gingival hyperplasia. Gingiva appears swollen and
red. False gingival pocket can also occur.

Wegener's Granulomatosis

Focal or diffuse gingival swelling can occur. It is characterized by epithelial proliferation and dense inflammatory
cell infiltration.

Carcinoma of the Gingiva

It is manifested as an area of ulceration, which may be a purely erosive lesion and may exhibit an exophytic, granular or verrucous type of growth. In some patients, the first symptom may be loosening of the teeth. It quickly spreads from the gingiva to alveolar bone below. The proximity of the underlying periosteum and bone usually invites early invasion of these structures (Fig. 15.16).

Radiologically, three types of bone destruction, i.e. permeated type (bone destruction with ill defined margins. Permeated means permeation of water into sand, with ragged ill defined borders. It also destroys the mandibular canal), moth eaten type (resembles moth eaten image with remnants of bony fragments) and pressure type (dish out

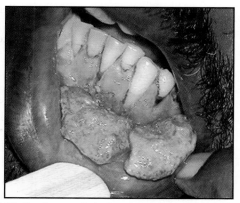

Fig. 15.16: Carcinoma of gingiva presenting as exophytic growth

concavity appearance with relatively smooth margins). Rarefaction with remnants of small bony fragment .

Localized lesions, of less than 3 cm in diameter, were cured in 80 percent of the cases; but the lesions over 5 cm in diameter had a poor outlook.

PERIODONTAL DISEASES

Periodontal Pockets

It can be gingival pocket (relative or false) (formed by gingival enlargement, without destruction of the underlying periodontal tissues), periodontal pocket (absolute or true) (destruction of the supporting periodontal tissue; progressive pocket deepening leads to destruction of the supporting periodontal tissues and loosening and exfoliation of the teeth), suprabony pocket (supracrestal or supra-alveolar) - in it, bottom of the pocket is coronal to the underlying alveolar bone) and infrabony (intrabony, subcrestal or intra-alveolar) (in it, bottom of the pocket is apical to the level of the adjacent alveolar bone)

Gingival bleeding or/and suppuration, tooth mobility and diastema formation may be present. In some cases, pus may be expressed by applying digital pressure. Patient may complain of localized pain or deep pain in the bone. When explored with a probe, the inner aspect of the periodontal pocket is generally painful (Fig. 15.17). There may be bluish red, thickened marginal gingiva and a bluish red vertical zone from the gingival margin to the alveolar mucosa.

Pockets are not detected on radiograph as they are soft tissue changes. Gutta percha points or caliberated silver

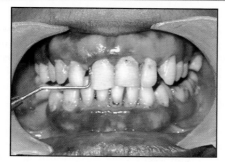

Fig. 15.17: Chronic periodontitis showing periodontal pockets

points can be used, with a radiograph, to assist in determining the level of attachment of the periodontal pocket.

Periodontitis

It is the most common type of periodontal infection, which results from an inflammatory reaction initiated in the gingiva with consequent spread to the supporting structures of the tooth.

Adult Periodontitis

It is also called as 'slowly progressive periodontitis', 'chronic adult periodontitis' and 'chronic inflammatory periodontitis'.

It is caused by local factors (plaque, calculus and poor oral hygiene) and systemic disease (diabetes mellitus, hormonal alteration or immunologic defect can accelerate periodontal diseases).

It can be mild periodontitis (attachment loss of 2 to 4 mm, minimum furcation invasion and little tooth mobility) moderate periodontitis (4 to 7 mm of probing attachment loss, early to moderate furcation invasion and slight to moderate tooth mobility) and severe periodontitis (probing attachment loss of 7 mm or more, with significant furcation invasion often through and through, with excessive tooth mobility).

It is usually painless, but sometimes exposed root may be sensitive to heat and cold, in absence of caries. Areas of localized deep pain, sometimes radiating deep into the jaws are established. The characteristic finding in it is gingival inflammation, which results from accumulation of plaque and loss of periodontal attachment (Fig. 15.18). The gingiva is slightly or moderately swollen and exhibits alteration in color from pale to magenta (Fig. 15.19). There is also loss of

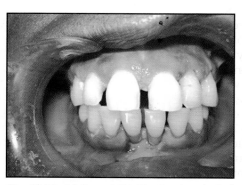

Fig. 15.18: Adults periodontitis showing gingival recession in lower anterior region

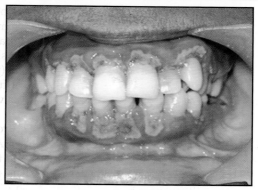

Fig. 15.19: Adults periodontitis showing gingival
recession and gingival inflammation

stippling and gingival bleeding, which may be either spontaneous or easily provoked.

There is presence of pocket with variable pocket depth. Both, horizontal and angular bone loss can be found. Tooth mobility is found in advanced cases, where bone loss has been considerable. Teeth give off a rather dull sound when tapped with a metal instrument.

Gingival recession is a common phenomenon in later stages of disease, which may expose the cementum (Fig. 15.20).

Radiologically there is blunting of the alveolar crest due to beginning of bone resorption. Loss of corticated interdental crestal margin, the bone edges become irregular or blunted. Widening of the periodontal ligament space and

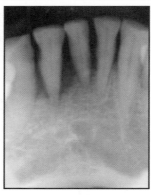

Fig. 15.20: Horizontal and vertical bone loss seen lower anterior region in adults periodontitis

localized or generalized loss of alveolar supporting bone. Bone loss may occur in horizontal, vertical or sometimes, in furcation area. Scaling and curettage can be done (Figs 15.19 to 15.24).

Rapidly Progressive Periodontitis

Microorganisms responsible are Actinobacillus actinomy-cetemcomitans, bacteroides gingivalis etc. Altered chemotactic response to neutrophils has been reported in some cases.

Rate of destruction is rapid over a period of time, as compared to slowly progressive periodontitis. Gingiva is acutely inflamed, often proliferated, ulcerated and fiery red (Fig. 15.25). Bleeding may occur spontaneously, or on slight

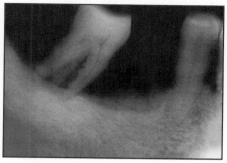

Fig. 15.21: Periodontitis showing furcation involvement and severe bone loss in posterior region

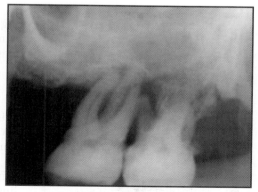

Fig. 15.22: Osseous defect seen upper posterior region

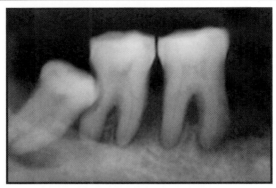

Fig. 15.23: Floating teeth appearance in severe periodontitis

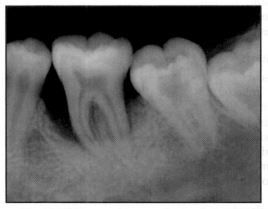

Fig. 15.24: Bony pocket seen distal to first molar

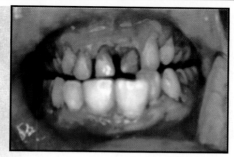

Fig. 15.25: Rapidly progressing periodontitis gingival enlargement and fiery red in color

provocation. In some cases, gingiva appears pink and free of inflammation; but in spite of this, deep pockets can be revealed on probing.

It is managed by antibiotics.

Juvenile Periodontitis

It is also called as 'periodontosis'. It is an autosomal recessive and X linked character. It is an aggressive, but uncommon form of periodontitis found in children and young adults.

It is a disease of the periodontium, occurring in an otherwise healthy adolescent and is characterized by a rapid loss of alveolar bone about one or more teeth of the permanent dentition.

It occur due to inherited defect in neutrophilic chemotactic function, which affects the ability of polymorphonuclear leukocytes to phagocytose and degranulate, thus impairing the host resistance.

The most striking feature is the lack of clinical inflammation, despite the presence of deep periodontal pockets. Initial complain is mobility and pathological drifting of first molars and incisors. Presence of deep pockets with secondary inflammation may occur.

Deep, dull radiating pain may occur with mastication, due to irritation of the supporting structures by mobile teeth and impacted food. Periodontal abscess may form at this stage and regional lymph node enlargement may occur. Rapid and typically angular loss of alveolar bone occurs, which may progress to tooth loss.

Radiologically vertical loss of alveolar bone around the first molars and incisors. Sometimes, bone loss may be generalized. There is an arc shaped loss of alveolar bone, extending from the distal surface of the second premolars to the mesial surface of second molars.

It is managed by standard periodontal therapy and antibiotic therapy.

Necrotizing Ulcerative Periodontitis

It occurs after repeated, long term episodes of acute necrotizing ulcerative gingivitis. Inflammatory infiltrate in the lesions of ANUG can extend to the underlying bone, resulting in a deep crater like osseous lesion most often located in the interdental area. There is a presence of deep interdental osseous crater but deep conventional pockets are not found, because the ulcerative and necrotizing character of the gingival lesion destroys the junctional epithelium the removing the mechanism of pocket deepening (Fig. 15.26).

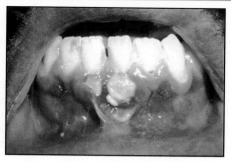

Fig. 15.26: Necrotizing ulcerative periodontitis characterized by ulceration in lower anterior region

As the patient may have underlying predisposing factors, it should be treated in consultation with a physician.

Tooth Mobility

Tooth has a slight degree of physiologic mobility, which varies from different teeth and at different times of the day. Mobility beyond the physiologic range is termed as abnormal or pathologic mobility.

It is caused by trauma from occlusion, loss of tooth support, extension of inflammation, osteomyelitis or jaw tumor, may also increase tooth mobility.

Radiologically there is a widening of periodontal ligament space and a single root may develop an hourglass shape (Fig. 15.27). Widening occurs as a result of resorption of root and alveolar bone. Lamina dura will be broad and hazy in density.

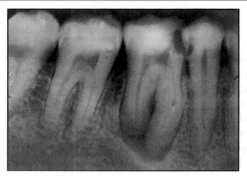

Fig. 15.27: Angular bone loss with furcation involvement seen with first molar

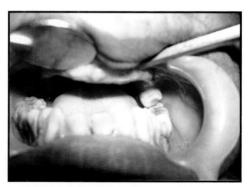

Fig. 15.28: Papillon-Lefevre syndrome presented as showing generalized recession and severe destruction of bone

Papillon-Lefevre Syndrome

It is an autosomal recessive and inherited disorder. It is a triad of:

- Hyperkeratosis of palms of the hand and soles of feet.
- Extensive prepubertal destruction of the periodontal bone supporting the dentition, usually extensive generalized horizontal bone loss (Fig. 15.28).
- Calcification of dura.

There is reddened, scaly, rough palms and soles, inflamed gingivae and horizontal bone destruction. It usually begins after eruption of the primary second molars. Loss of entire primary dentition by the age of 5 years and loss of secondary dentition by the age of 20 years. Gingival swelling and severe halitosis.

TMJ Disorders

It is a unique joint in which translatory as well as rotational movements are possible and where both the ends of bone articulate, in the same plane, with that of other bone (Fig. 16.1). It is also called as ginglymodiarthrodial type of joint, meaning that it has a relatively sliding type of movement between bony surfaces, in addition to hinge movement, common to diarthodial joint.

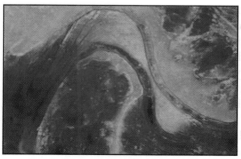

Fig. 16.1: Sagittal cross-section showing normal disc positioning of the TMJ

DEVELOPMENTAL DISORDERS OF THE TMJ

Hypoplasia of Condyle

It can be unilateral or bilateral. It is cause by chromosomal anomalies, achondroplasia, mandibulofacial dysostosis, progeria, Larsen's syndrome, Pierre robin syndrome, radiation to fetus, Mobius syndrome, hypothyroidism and hypopituitarism, vitamin A deficiency, trauma, infection and rheumatoid arthritis.

In unilateral type on unaffected side, there is elongation of the body of mandible and flat appearance of the face. Mandible shifts towards the affected side on opening. Eruption may be delayed in case of hypoplasia of the condyle.

When there is bilateral arrest of condylar growth, there is usually a symmetrical lack of growth of the mandible which results in *micrognathia* with the chin retruded to about the level of hyoid bone. Disturbance of eruption and malocclusion occurs.

Radiologically a short condylar process is seen. The condyle tends to assume a more posterior position. The neck of the condyle is slender (Fig. 16.2). There may be proportionate shortening of the ramus and body on the affected side and the bone tends to be smaller than the opposite side. There is a shallow sigmoid and antegonial notch with impacted teeth. In cases of bilateral under development, all the above features plus bilateral antegonial notching is seen.

Surgical, orthodontic and prosthetic procedures give functional and cosmetic improvement.

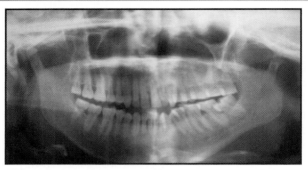

Fig. 16.2: Hypoplasia of left condyle (*Courtesy*: Dr Ashok L, Professor and Head, Oral Medicine and Radiology, Bapuji Dental College and Hospital, Davanagere, India)

Hyperplasia of the Condyle

It is caused by hemi facial hypertrophy, chondroma, osteochondroma or osteoma of condyle, fibrous dysplasia, Paget's disease, Klinefelter syndrome, gigantism, and acromegaly.

In unilateral type there is slowly developing distraction and enlargement of TMJ. Progressive enlargement of the mandible occurs. There is facial asymmetry and shifting of the midline of chin to the unaffected side, with resulting cross bite, or open bite on the affected side.

In bilateral type mandible is larger and more forward than the maxilla. Mandibular teeth are anterior to the maxillary teeth (anterior cross bite). Obtuse mandibular angle and the sigmoid notch form an arc of a larger circle.

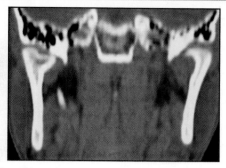

Fig. 16.3: Coronal section showing enlarged right head of the condyle (*Courtesy:* Dr Avinash Kshar and Dr Umarji, Government Dental College and Hospital, Mumbai)

Radiologically the ramus and body of the affected side of mandible are larger. The vertical ramus is increased in vertical depth as well as in its antero-posterior diameter. It results in prevention of occlusion of the posterior teeth. The body of the bone is also elongated and enlarged in some cases. The condylar enlargement is sometimes symmetrically distributed throughout the whole process (Fig. 16.3). The angle of the jaw is right angle in some cases and is more obtuse than normal in some cases. The articular eminence is shallower than the opposite normal side, with the distal surface slightly evacuated (Fig. 16.3).

Orthognathic surgery to improve esthetics and function of mandible.

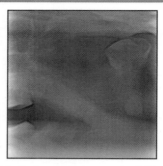

Fig. 16.4: Radiographic image of a bifid condyle

DOUBLE CONDYLE

It is caused by persistence of the well vascularized fibrous tissue septa, which is normally present in the condylar cartilage during embryonal and early postnatal life. Possible rupture of some of the blood vessels contained within the septa might impair the ossification of the condyle so as to cause a bifid development of the condylar head.

There is limitation of opening of mouth, a small lateral deviation. Lateral movement is limited. Radio-logically double mandibular condyle (Fig. 16.4). There may be two separate glenoid fossa.

It is managed by surgical treatment.

DEGENERATIVE JOINT DISEASE

Osteoarthritis

It is also called as *'osteoarthrosis'* or *'degenerative arthritis'*. It is primarily a disorder of movable joints characterized by deterioration and abrasion of the articular cartilage with formation of new bone at the joint surface. There is destruction of the soft tissue component of the joint and subsequent erosion with hypertrophic changes in bone. There is breakdown of the connective tissue covering of the condyle, articular eminence and the disk.

It is common in many joints, but it is not frequently found in TMJ. Unilateral pain over the joint, which may be sensitive to palpation. Pain on movements or biting, which may limit mandibular function. There is deviation of the jaw towards the affected side and stiffness of the joint. There is limitation of jaw movements, which becomes increasingly apparent with function. Early signs may progress to spasm of the masticatory muscles resulting in stiffness and locking of the jaw.

Radiologically there is evidence of erosion of condyle on a radiograph occurs on an average, 6 months after the onset of TMJ pain. Density is increased as a result of sclerosis. Small crescent like excavation appears at the superior aspect of the condyle just behind the point of articular contact. This is followed by wooly appearance, with spreading of rarefaction in the bone beneath the articular surface. Fully developed lesions are saucer shaped on PA view. This is also called as the destructive phase (Fig. 16.5).

Eminence is flattened or almost removed and anterior half of the superior convex surface of the condyle is converted into a flat plane. Mandibular fossa is enlarged and becomes shallow. Development of lipping (shell like extension) on the anterior borders. There is also *osteophyte formation (Fig. 16.6), Ely's cyst (*small radiolucent areas are usually

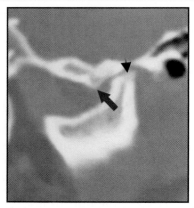

Fig. 16.5: Sagittal reconstruction showing flattening of the head of condyle superiorly and articular eminence posteroinferiorly

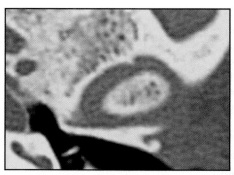

Fig. 16.6: Axial section, osteophyte of glenoid fossa (*Courtesy*: Dr Avinash Kshar and Dr Umarji, Government Dental College and Hospital, Mumbai)

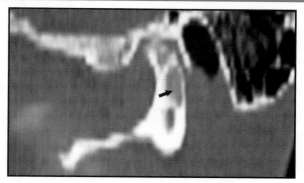

Fig. 16.7: Ely's cyst (arrow) presented as a well defined radiolucent cavity in the condyle (*Courtesy*: Dr Avinash Kshar and Dr Umarji, Government Dental College and Hospital, Mumbai

less sharply defined and may have slightly irregular borders. These areas are regarded as cystic and are given the name '*Ely's cyst*') (Fig. 16.7).

It is managed by heat therapy, diathermy and ultrasonic. Muscle exercises, injection of local anesthetic in TMJ. Other treatment modalities are analgesics, anti-inflammatory drugs, tranquilizers and muscle relaxants, intra-articular injection of corticosteroids.

INFLAMMATORY DISORDERS OF THE JOINT

Rheumatoid Arthritis

It is a debilitating systemic disease of unknown origin, characterized by progressive involvement of the joint, particularly bilateral involvement of large joints.

It results from systemic infection, which evokes an inflammatory response within the joint.

In typical cases, small joints of fingers and toes are the first to be affected. Symptoms include bilateral stiffness, crepitus, tenderness and swelling over the joint. Fever, malaise, fatigue, weight loss, pain and stiffness in the limb are also evident.

TMJ involvement can be acute or chronic. In acute cases, there is bilateral stiffness, deep seated pain, tenderness on palpation and swelling over the joint. There is limitation in opening of mouth. In chronic cases, crepitus is the most frequent finding. Functional disturbances like deviation on opening and inability to perform lateral excursions are common.

There is flattening of the head of the condyle. Erosion of the condyle can be seen (Fig. 16.8). As the disease continues,

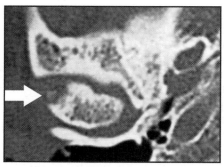

Fig. 16.8: Axial section, erosion of the head of condyle seen on the lateral side (*Courtesy*: Dr Avinash Kshar and Dr Umarji, Government Dental College and Hospital, Mumbai)

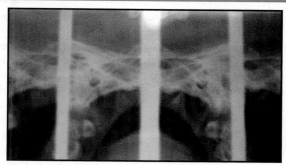

Fig. 16.9: Sharpened pencil appearance seen in the case of arthritis (*Courtesy:* Dr Amit Parate, Lecturer, Oral Medicine and Radiology, GDCH, Nagpur, India)

the condylar outline becomes increasingly irregular and ragged. In most severe cases, condyle may be completely resorbed, resulting in loss of vertical support and anterior open bite. In advanced stages, erosion of anterior and posterior condylar surface at the attachment of the synovial lining occurs, which may resemble a 'sharpened pencil' or 'mouth piece of flute' (Fig. 16.9).

Adequate rest to the joint, soft diet is advocated. Treatment should be given for suppression of the active process, preservation of function and prevention of deformities. *Intraarticular corticosteroid injections and non-steroidal anti-inflammatory drugs should be given.*

Infective Arthritis

It is also called as *'septic arthritis'*. It may be acute or chronic.

It is caused by direct spread of organisms like staphylococci, streptococci, pneumococci and gonococci, from an infected mastoid process, tympanic cavity or via blood. It may also be caused by trauma directly to the joint or infection from a maxillary molar and parotid gland.

In accute phase there is severe pain on jaw movement, with an inability to place the teeth in occlusion, due to presence of infection in the joint. Redness and swelling over the joint. Infection of both the compartments of the joint also occurs. Tender cervical lymph nodes on the side of infection. This helps to distinguish septic arthritis from other temporomandibular joint disorders.

Chronic type may follow an acute infection. One joint is affected, but bilateral involvement can occur. Ankylosis of the joint or facial asymmetry, (if the growth centers are involved) may occur.

Radiologically in acute cases joint space may be increased by inflammatory distension in early infective period. There is an increase in width of the joint space. There is hazy appearance in radiographs. In chronic cases, there may be peripheral condensing osteitis and approximation of the joint surface, as the articular cartilage is eroded. There may be frank bone destruction. A small cup shaped excavation on the anterior face of the condyle, having a smooth or irregular base is seen (Figs 16.10 and 16.11). In rare cases whole of the condyle may be lost with varying amount of eminence.

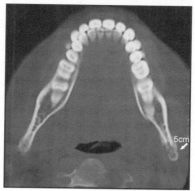

Fig. 16.10: Destruction of the condyle occurring in infective arthritis (*Courtesy*: Dr Bhaskar Patle, Lecturer, SPDC Wardha)

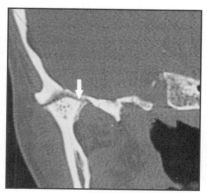

Fig. 16.11: Coronal section showing erosion of head of condyle superiorly and glenoid fossa (*Courtesy*: Dr Avinash Kshar and Dr Umarji, Government Dental College and Hospital, Mumbai)

It is managed by rest to the joint and limitation of movements. Liquid diet, appropriate antibiotics and analgesics should be given.

TRAUMATIC DISORDERS OF TMJ

Condylar Fracture

It can be intracapsular and extracapsular.

It can occurs due to indirect violence and parade ground fracture (if the blow is sustained centrally on the chin then there is a possibility of bilateral fracture of the condyle. This commonly occurs when a soldier faints on a parade ground and hence named as 'parade ground fracture).

Unilateral fracture—pain on the affected side; it is increased when movement is attempted. Patient complains that his teeth do not occlude in the normal fashion. Inability to bring the jaw forward. Small localized swelling over the injured TMJ. There is bleeding from the ear on the affected side which results from laceration of the anterior wall of the external auditory meatus. Tenderness may be present over the condylar area. Occasional crepitus and deviation of the mandible to the affected side. There is gagging of the ipsilateral molar teeth.

Bilateral fracture—all the above signs plus variable degree of gagging of the occlusion on the molar teeth. Overall mandibular movements are more restricted, than in unilateral fracture (Fig. 16.12). Mandible is displaced forwards in case of bilateral fracture

In fracture dislocation all the above findings plus a definite absence of condyle in the glenoid fossa. It can be

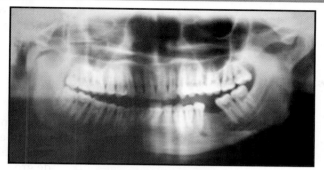

Fig. 16.12: Bilateral condylar fracture
with loss of occlusal contact

unilateral dislocation (if the condylar head is dislocated
medially and all edema has subsided due to passage of
time, it may be possible to observe a characteristic 'hollow'
over the region of the condylar head), *bilateral dislocation* (if
there is a bilateral dislocation, then there is an anterior open
bite present) and *central dislocation* (it is a rare type of injury
which is usually severe and forces the condyle into the
cranial cavity through the floor of the articular fossa. It is
termed as central dislocation of the TMJ).

Radiologically displaced condylar fracture is well
demonstrated on AP and lateral projection (Fig. 16.13). Non-
displaced fracture is well seen on AP view.

The fracture line is often transverse but usually oblique,
starting in the base of the mandibular notch and passing
slightly or even markedly downwards (Fig. 16.14). In
absence of any displacement, it is difficult to visualize such

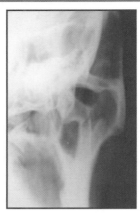

Fig. 16.13: Transorbital view of the condylar
fracture showing medial displacement

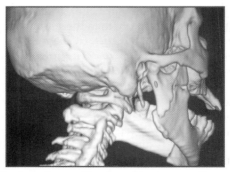

Fig. 16.14: Fracture of coronoid and condylar process with symphysis fracture (*Courtesy*: Dr Amit Parate, Lecturer, Oral Medicine and Radiology, GDC Nagpur, India)

fractures. In the lateral projection there is often no evidence of any fracture line; but when the posterior margin of the ramus is followed, a sudden step is seen. It is managed by immobilization.

Ankylosis

Ankylosis, a Greek word which means *'stiff joint'*. It is an abnormal immobility and consolidation of the joint.

It can be *true (intra-articular) or false (extra-articular), bony or fibrous, partial or complete.*

It is caused by fibrosis, epilepsy, brain tumor, bulbar paralysis and cerberovascular accidents, and osteochondroma.

There is pain and trismus which is directly related to the duration of ankylosis. Depending upon the duration, there may poor oral hygiene, carious teeth and periodontal problems malocclusion.

In unilateral type mouth opening is impossible (Fig. 16.15), but the patient may be able to produce several mms of interincisal opening. Asymmetry of the face with fullness on the affected side and relative flattening on the unaffected side (Fig. 16.16). In unilateral ankylosis, patient's face is deviated towards the affected side. The chin is retracted on the affected side and slightly bypasses the midline. Slight gliding movement towards the affected side. Cross bite is present.

In bilateral face is symmetrical with micrognathia. There is bird face appearance (Fig. 16.17). With bilateral ankylosis, neither protrusive nor lateral movements are possible.

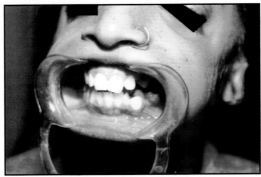

Fig. 16.15: Ankylosis of TMJ showing no opening of the mouth

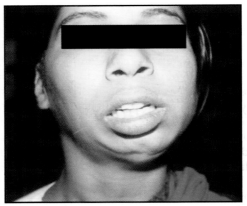

Fig. 16.16: Unilateral ankylosis showing deviation of
mandible towards affected side

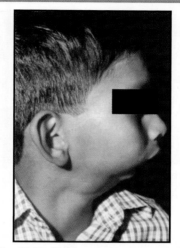

Fig. 16.17: Bird face appearance seen in bilateral ankylosis of the TMJ

In bony ankylosis, there is no pain but in case of fibrous ankylosis there is pain. Due to long standing ankylosis, atrophy or fibrosis of muscles of mastication may result. In case of congenital ankylosis, there is difficulty of introducing the nipple into the mouth of newborn infants.

Radiologically there is transverse or oblique dark line, irregular in outline, crossing the mass of dense bone (Fig. 16.18). When a dark line is present, the possibility of fibrous ankylosis is more. The ramus is vertical and the angle is reduced in size. The body of the jaw is short. The condyle may retain its normal shape, but it can be replaced by

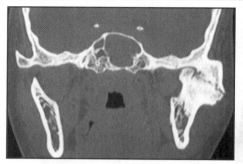

Fig. 16.18: Coronal section showing irregular articular surfaces with lost normal joint space, central part of the head of condyle fused with glenoid fossa (*Courtesy*: Dr Avinash Kshar and Dr Umarji, Government Dental College and Hospital, Mumbai)

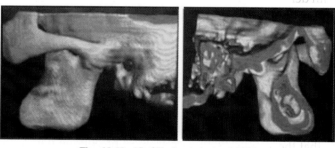

Fig. 16.19: 3D CT of ankylosis of TMJ

shapeless mass of bone, which finds attachment to the base of skull above and to the base of neck of condyle below (Fig. 16.19). There is deformity of the ramus and body of the mandible in some cases of fibrous ankylosis. In bony

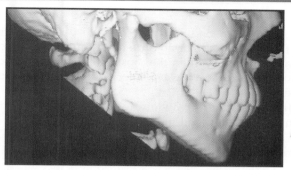

Fig. 16.20: Ankylosis of TMJ (*Courtesy*: Dr Bhaskar Patle)

ankylosis joint space is completely or partially obliterated with dense sclerotic bone (Fig. 16.20). Sometimes, large mass of new bone may be seen, radiographically obscuring the condyle and joint space.

Prominent antegonial notch on the affected side of mandible, along with inferior arching of the mandibular body (secondary to isotonic contraction of the depressor muscles). Bone may form around the neck of the condyle and becomes continuous with the base of the skull. Considerable destruction of bone may precede bony ankylosis.

The greater part of the condyle may have been destroyed so that the sigmoid or mandibular notch is approximated to the base of the skull. The neck of the condyle, if not completely hidden by the mass of new bon, appears to be shortened; so that the mandibular notch is nearer the zygomatic process than normal. No translation of condyle head during opening.

It is managed by condylectomy, *gap arthroplasty.*

DISLOCATION

It results when condyle is forcefully displaced anteriorly (by failure of muscular co-ordination) out of the articular fossa but remains within the capsule of joint. The direction of condyle is almost always anterior, beyond the articular eminence.

It can be anterior dislocation, posterior dislocation, central dislocation and medial or lateral dislocation.

Anterior Dislocation

In acute dislocation, there is a history of injury, gagging of molar teeth and anterior open bite. Patient has great difficulty in swallowing and saliva drools over the chin. Pain in the region of temporal fossa and there is a depression where the condylar head is normally situated. The mandible is postured forward and movement is extremely limited. The condyle becomes locked anterior to the articular eminence and is prevented from sliding back by muscular spasm. When unilateral dislocation occurs, the teeth will be gagged posteriorly on the side of dislocation and the chin will be deviated towards the normal side. Radiologically there is a wide variation in anterior condylar movements. Condyle is locked in front of the articular disc.

Central Dislocation

The head of the condyle is forced through the floor of the articular fossa, into the floor of middle cranial fossa. In this case, there may be damage to the articular surface of the condyle and fracture of the neck. Neurological signs like the cerebral contusion, facial nerve paralysis, deafness and bleeding from the ear may also be present.

Posterior Dislocation

It results from severe injury, which forces the mandible backwards, so that the condyle penetrates the tympanic plate of the temporal bone. When the upward and backward thrust is applied to the chin, posterior dislocation occurs. There may be tenderness over the affected TMJ, limited mouth opening, anterior open bite and laterognathism. Radiologically, the anterior portion of the articular fossa is empty and the condyle is seen too far posteriorly.

It is managed by traction and immobilization for 2 weeks. Sometimes, open reduction may be required.

SUBLUXATION (HYPERMOBILITY)

It is the unilateral or bilateral positioning of the condyle anterior to the articular eminence, with repositioning to normal accomplished physiologic activity. It is self-reducing incomplete dislocation, which generally follows stretching of the capsule and ligaments.

It is caused by *long continuous opening of mouth, oral surgical procedures, osteoarthritis, psychiatric problem*, and use of *phenothiazine*.

Cracking noise, temporary locking of the condyle and immobilization of the jaw is present. Patient describes weakness of the joint while yawning. Pain is associated with last few millimeters of mouth opening. The condyle may get locked when the mouth is opened widely and upon

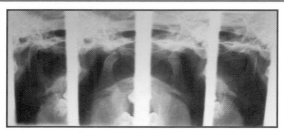

Fig. 16.21: Subluxation of TMJ observed on panoramic radiograph (*Courtesy:* Dr Tapasya Karamore, Lecturer Department of Oral Medicine and Radiology, VSPM Dental College and Research Centre, Nagpur, India)

closing, it will return with a jumping motion, accompanied by a sound caused by movement of the condyle over the articular eminence. On palpation *'click'* on opening and sliding of condyle over the articular eminence, are common.

Radiologically excessive excursion of the condyle from rest position to the position when jaw is opened wide (Fig. 16.21).

Here the objective is achieved by shrinking the capsule by a sclerosing agent, which will cause fibrosis of the capsule.

DISC DISLOCATION

If the posterior border of the disc becomes thinner and the retrodiscal lamina and collateral ligament become more elongated, the disc can slip anteriorly through the discal space. This is known as disc dislocation, as there is loss of contact between the articular surfaces of the condyle and the disc.

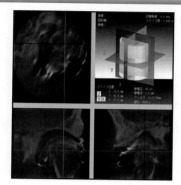

Fig. 16.22: Double contrast CBCT arthrography—it demonstrated anterior displacement of the disc without perforation and dilation of the superior joint space. Also, demonstrated multiple loculi in the anterior region of the joint space. (*Courtesy*: Kazuya Honda, DDS, PhD Department of Radiology, Nihon University School of Dentistry 1-8-13 Kanda-Surugadai, Chiyoda-ku, Tokyo 101-8310, Japan)

Disc dislocation with reduction—during the disc dislocation, the condyle may articulate on the retrodiscal tissue and may cause pain. On physical examination, the joint is tender and reciprocal clicking is heard. The jaw deviated towards the side of the click, till the click occurs and then returns to the midline.

Disc dislocation patient who experiences repeated disc dislocations with reduction may further elongate discal ligament and retrodiscal lamina. Often, elasticity of the retrodiscal lamina is lost. If the condyle moves forward but the disc is not returned to its normal relationship between the condyle and fossa, a condition known as dislocation without reduction occurs (Fig. 16.22). It is also called as closed lock. There is joint pain, limited opening, previous clicking with intermittent locking and sensation of something in the joint. There is joint tenderness with deviation towards the affected side. Terminal stretching produces increased joint pain.

Disc Displacement with Perforation

There is joint pain, clicking with intermittent locking and closed lock. There is also limited opening. Crepitus and grinding noise. There is also joint tenderness.

Radiologically they are not diagnostic; except in case of perforation of the disc, where there is evidence of degenerative changes in the joint. Arthrogram is useful in studying the changes.

Adhesions

The movements between healthy articular surfaces occur without friction. Changes in the articular surfaces and synovial fluid can drastically change this frictionless system. This sticking of articular surfaces has been called as *adhesion*.

Adhesions can occur in either superior or inferior joint space and can occur with or without disc derangement (Figs 16.23 and 16.24). Adhesion can begin after prolonged static loading of the joint. The patient wakes up with limited jaw movement. As the patient attempts to move the mandible, a single click is felt (representing freeing of adhesion) and then, the normal range movement is restored. The click only occurs once and can not be repeated without prolonged period of static loading.

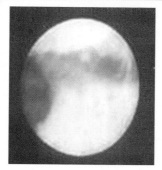

Fig. 16.23: Arthroscopic observation - band like fibrous adhesion was observed in the posterior articular cavity (*Courtesy*: Kazuya Honda, DDS, PhD Department of Radiology, Nihon University School of Dentistry 1-8-13 Kanda-Surugadai, Chiyoda-ku, Tokyo 101-8310, Japan)

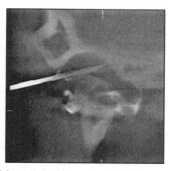

Fig. 16.24: CBCT frontal double contrast image. The disc was slightly medially displacement, and adhesion was partially observed. (*Courtesy:* Kazuya Honda, DDS, PhD Department of Radiology, Nihon University School of Dentistry 1-8-13 Kanda-Surugadai, Chiyoda-ku, Tokyo 101-8310, Japan)

NEOPLASTIC DISORDERS

Benign Tumors

Benign tumors reported are osteoma and osteochondroma. There is stiffness of the joint with facial asymmetry. Deviation of mandible on the affected side. Disordered occlusion, little movement of the condyle on palpation. Restricted movements of TMJ.

Radiographically

There is bony mass protruding from the condyle.

Management is surgical excision of the tumor and orthodontic treatment, to re-establish the occlusion.

Malignant tumors

Intrinsic

Arises from the bone of the condyle, articular fossa and the joint capsule or the articular disc. It includes chondro-sarcoma and synovial sac sarcoma (Figs 16.25 and 16.26).

Extrinsic

The tumors which extend from outside of TMJ, e.g. neoplasm of the parotid gland.

Pain on full opening of the mouth and diminished hearing. Swelling of the TMJ. The tumor may be fixed to deep structures. Deviation of the mandible to the unaffected side. There is also malocclusion.

It can be treated by surgery, chemotherapy, radiotherapy and combination therapy

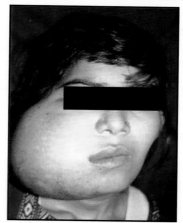

Fig. 16.25: Chondrosarcoma of condyle
showing huge swelling on the left side

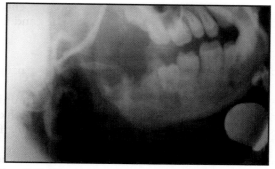

Fig. 16.26: Chondrosarcoma showing destruction of condyle

MISCELLANEOUS DISORDERS

Synovial Chondromatosis

It is a benign chronic progressive metaplasia that will not resolve spontaneously. Although it is non-neoplastic, it may resemble a malignant condition histologically.

It denotes the condition whereby a cartilaginous focus develops within the synovial membrane of the joint. Eventually, they are detached from the affected membrane and become cartilaginous mobile bodies within the joint cavity.

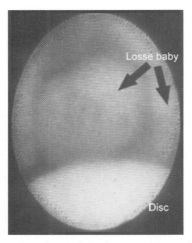

Fig. 16.27: Arthroscopy observation—the image shows the loose circular bodies of a tumor in the joint space, the patient was diagnosed as having synovial chondromatosis. (*Courtesy*: Kazuya Honda, DDS, PhD Department of Radiology, Nihon University School of Dentistry 1-8-13 Kanda-Surugadai, Chiyoda-ku, Tokyo 101-8310, Japan)

Many of these cartilaginous foci then undergo calcification. These joint bodies acquire a perichondrium, which enables them to grow by proliferation of chondrocytes. Trauma may be a predisposing factor, others factors are malocclusion, occlusal habits, subluxation or tension sites.

There is facial pain, limitation of motion and deviation towards the affected side. Crepitus, preauricular swelling, enlarged joint with effusion and local tenderness.

Radiologically intrajoint and perijoint densities are noted (Fig. 16.27).

These bodies, if symptomatic, should be removed.

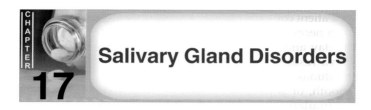

17 Salivary Gland Disorders

DEVELOPMENTAL DISORDERS OF SALIVARY GLAND

Aberrancy

It is defined as that situation in which the salivary gland tissue develops at a site where it is not normally found. It is also called as ectopic salivary gland.

The aberrancy of the salivary gland tissue represents only an extreme example of the condition known as the *'developmental lingual mandibular salivary gland depression'*. It is the developmental inclusion of the glandular tissue within or more commonly, adjacent to the lingual surface of the body of the mandible, in a deep well circumscribed depression. It was first described by Stafne in 1942 and hence referred to as 'Stafne's cyst'.

Ectopic salivary gland tissue has been reported to occur in the gingiva, where it may be described as *'gingival salivary gland choristoma'*.

Aplasia and Hypoplasia

Aplasia or agenesis is the congenital absence of the salivary gland (Fig.17.1). It was first described by *Gruber* in 1885.

Patient complains of xerostomia, which may be so severe as to necessitate the constant sipping of water throughout the day and particularly, during meal times. The lack of saliva results in rampant dental caries and early loss of deciduous and permanent teeth. Oral mucosa appears dry, smooth, or sometimes pebbly and shows a tendency for accumulation of debris. Patients exhibit characteristic cracking of lips and fissuring of the corners of mouth. Hypoplasia of salivary glands is rare but hypoplasia of parotid gland has been reported to be present with Melkerson Rosenthal syndrome.

Institution of scrupulous oral hygiene in an attempt to decrease dental caries and preserve the teeth as long as possible.

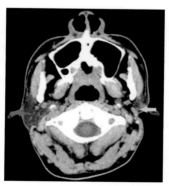

Fig. 17.1: Hypoplasia of the unilateral parotid gland (Plain CT). Size of the left parotid gland (yellow arrow) is remarkably smaller compared with normal size of the right parotid gland (red arrow) (*Courtesy:* Dr M Shizumu)

HYPERPLASIA OF SALIVARY GLAND

It is caused by endocrine disorders and menopause, gout, diabetes mellitus, Sjögren's syndrome, Waldenstrom macro-globulinemia, aglossia-adactylia syndrome, Heerfordt's syndrome and Felty's syndrome and hepatic disease, starvation, alcoholism, inflammation, benign lympho-epithelial lesion, adiposity, hyperthermia, oligomenorrhea and certain drugs.

Palatal gland hyperplasia appears as small localized swelling of varying size, measuring from several millimeters to 1 cm, usually on the hard palate or at junction of hard and soft palate. The lesion has an intact surface and is firm, sessile and normal in color.

Atresia

It is the congenital occlusion or absence of one or two major salivary gland ducts. The newborn infant presents, within 2 or 3 days of life, with submandibular swelling on the affected side due to the presence of a retention cyst. It may produce a relatively severe xerostomia.

Developmental Salivary Gland Defect

It is also called as 'static bone cavity or cyst', 'Stafne's cyst or defect', 'lingual mandibular bone cavity' and 'latent bone cyst'. It is the developmental inclusion of glandular tissue within or more commonly, adjacent to the lingual surface of the body of mandible. It was recognized by Stafne in 1942.

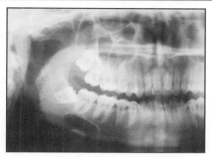

Fig. 17.2: Stafne's cystic cavity (*Courtesy:* Dr Tapasya Karamore, Lecturer, Oral Medicine and Radiology, VSPM Dental College and Research Center, Nagpur, India)

Radiologically round or ovoid radiolucency that will vary in size from 1 to 3 cm in diameter (Fig. 17.2). It is occasionally bilateral. It is well defined by dense radiopaque border that is the result of the rays passing tangentially through the relatively thick wall of depression.

OBSTRUCTIVE DISORDERS
Sialolithiasis

It is the also called as '*salivary gland stone*' or '*salivary gland calculus*'.

It is formation of calcific concretions within the parenchyma or ductal system of the major or minor salivary glands.

It is caused by *neurohumoral mechanism, metabolic mechanism*. It can be ductal sialoliths or glandular sialoliths.

Many patients complain of moderately severe pain and intermittent transient swelling during meals, which resolves after meals. As the calculus itself rarely blocks a duct

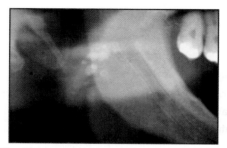

Fig. 17.3: Sialolithiasis of salivary gland showing stones as radiopacity

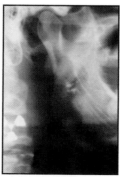

Fig. 17.4: Sialolith parotid gland 1 and 2-multiple calculi in midramus (*Courtesy:* of Dr. Enzio Rovigatti) Manual manipulation of stone within the duct

completely, the swelling subsides as salivary demand diminishes and as saliva seeps past the partial obstruction. Pus may exude from the duct orifice. The soft tissues surrounding the duct show a severe inflammatory reaction, which may appear as swelling, redness and tenderness.

Projection for submandibular duct stone is standard mandibular occlusal view and for parotid gland, periapical view in the buccal vestibule. Reduce the exposure to avoid burnout of sialoliths. Sialography is indicated when sialoliths are radiolucent. There is ductal dilatation caused by associated sialodochitis. The film usually shows contrast medium present behind the stone. They are almost radiopaque, so that even very small ones are visible in well made radiograph (Figs 17.3 to 17.5A and B). It is usually oval shaped and cylindrical with multiple layers of

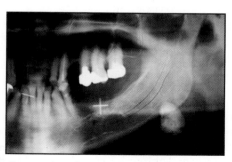

Fig. 17.5A: Panoramic radiograph showing sialolith in submandibular gland (*Courtesy:* of Dr. Enzio Rovigatti)

calcification. Smooth borders with even radiodensity. It may be solitary or multiple.

CYSTS OF SALIVARY GLAND
Mucocele

It is a term used to describe the swelling caused by pooling of saliva at the site of injured minor salivary gland.

It can be mucus *extravasation* (extravasation of mucus into the connective tissue) and mucus *retention* (obstruction of minor salivary gland duct which causes the backup of saliva).

Patient may complain of painless swelling which is frequently recurrent. The swelling may suddenly develop at meal time and may drain simultaneously at intervals. The mucocele may be only 1-2 mm in diameter, but is usually larger; majority of them being between 5 to 10 mm in diameter. Superficial cyst appears as bluish mass, as the thin overlying mucosa permits the pool of mucus fluid to absorb most of visible wave length of light. The swelling is round or oval and smooth. It is either soft or hard depending upon the tension in the fluid. It can not be emptied by digital pressure.

Ranula

It is derived from Latin word '*Rana tigerina*' i.e. frog belly. The term ranula is used for the mucoceles occurring in the floor of the mouth, in association with ducts of submandibular or sublingual glands. It can be *superficial and plunging types.*

They produce blue swelling like a frog's belly; hence it was given the term 'ranula' ('ranula' in Greek mean frog's belly). The overlying mucosa in normal in appearance. It develops as slowly enlarging painless mass on one side of the floor of mouth (Fig. 17.5B). When the swelling suddenly

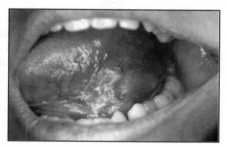

Fig. 17.5B: Ranula seen as bluish swelling one side in floor of mouth

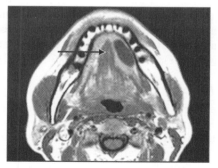

Fig. 17.6: Ranula T₁ weighted MR image shows lower signal intensity than that of muscles in the left sublingual region—arrow (*Courtesy:* Dr M Shizumu)

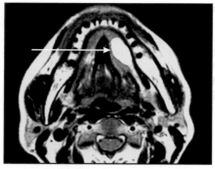

Fig. 17.7: Ranula T_2 weighted MR image of the same case. Note the remarkably high signal intensity of the lesion—arrow (*Courtesy:* M Shizumu)

grows it may be painful. Big ranula may cause difficulty in speech or eating. It is spherical or dome shaped with only top half is visible. It is soft and tends to fluctuant. It can not empty by pressure and is non-pulsatile. *Fluctuation and transillumination* tests are positive. On MRI it is visible as lower signal intensity on T_1 and high signal intensity on T_2 (Figs 17.6 and 17.7)

Plunging Ranula

When intrabuccal ranula has a cervical prolongation, it is called as deep or plunging ranula. It is derived from cervical sinus. Sometimes, plunging ranula herniated through the mylohyoid muscle and causes a swelling in suprahyoid or infrahyoid region. To inspect plunging ranula, bidigital palpation should be performed. On finger is placed inside the mouth on the ranula and the other finger is place on the swelling in the submandibular region. If pressure on the first finger causes sense of fluctuation on 2nd finger or vice versa, then it is plunging ranula.

They are best treated by surgical excision including a portion of the surrounding tissues.

Asymptomatic enlargement of the salivary gland Sialosis (sialadenosis)

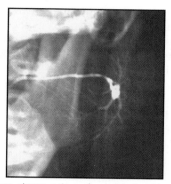

Fig. 17.8: Sialogram shows enlarged parotid gland in sialosis, however, peripheral ducts are normal (*Courtesy:* M Shizumu)

It is characterized by non-neoplastic non-inflammatory enlargement of the salivary gland. The enlargement is usually bilateral and may present a course of recurrent painless enlargement of gland (Fig. 17.8). The parotid gland is more frequently affected and more commonly affects the females. Swelling of the preauricular portion of the parotid gland is the most common symptom, but retromandibular portion of the gland may also be affected. The condition is found in association with systemic diseases especially cirrhosis, diabetes, ovarian and thyroid insufficiency, alcoholism and malnutrition. A characteristic alteration in the chemical constituents of saliva is a distinguishing feature of sialosis.

Allergic Sialadenitis

In some cases, it may not appear as a true hypersensitivity reaction but rather as a toxic or idiosyncratic reaction to drugs that cause a deceased salivary flow, resulting in secondary infection. Various drugs which have been reported to cause allergic sialoadentitis include sulfisoxazole, phenothiazines, iodine containing compounds, mercury, thiouracil and phenylbutazone.

The clinical appearance of allergic sialadenitis varies, but in most of the cases there is bilateral parotid gland enlargement following the administration of the drug. The enlargement may be painful and is usually associated with conjunctivitis and skin rashes. It is a self limiting disease and needs no treatment.

VIRAL INFECTION

Various viruses like paramyxovirus, cytomegalovirus, parainfluenza type-3 and coxsackie virus may infect salivary glands and cause its enlargement.

Mumps

It is an acute contagious viral infection, characterized chiefly by unilateral or bilateral swelling of the salivary glands. It mainly affects major salivary glands, but also affects the testis, meninges, pancreas, heart and mammary glands. It is also called as 'endemic parotitis'.

It is caused by paramyxovirus. It is preceded by onset of headache, chills, moderate fever, vomiting and pain below the ear which lasts for about one week. Both the parotid glands may involve simultaneously, but more commonly one parotid gland swells 24 to 48 hours after the other. It is then followed by sudden onset of salivary gland swelling which is firm somewhat rubbery or elastic and without purulent discharge from the salivary gland duct. The enlargement of parotid gland causes elevation of ear lobule and it produces pain upon mastication especially while eating sour food. Papilla on the opening of parotid duct is often puffy and reddened. Salivary amylase level is increased.

It is self-limiting, with salivary gland enlargement subsiding within a week.

Bacterial Infection

Bacterial infection of salivary gland may be recurrent and generally develops owing to spread of microorganisms from the oral flora along the excretory duct.

Acute Bacterial Sialadenitis

It is also called as 'acute suppurative parotitis.

It is caused by microorganisms, dehydration, malnutrition, cancer and surgical infections. Poor oral hygiene is an important contributory factor. Drugs like anti-

Parkinson's, diuretics and antihistaminic have been reported to be a contributory factor for acute bacterial sialadenitis.

It begins with the elevation of body temperature and sudden onset of pain at the angle of the jaw which is intense.

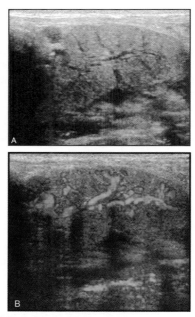

Figs 17.9A and B: Sonograms of acute sialadenitis of the submandibular gland scanned perpendicular to the mandibular plane (left side: cranial, right side: caudal). A: The left submandibular gland shows swelling, however, normal echo level. The black lines inside the gland are not dilated ducts, they are blood vessels; B: The gland shows increased vascularity (*Courtesy:* Dr M Shizumu)

Parotid gland is tender, enlarged and the overlying skin is warm and red (Figs 17.9A and B). The swelling usually causes elevation of the ear lobule and the overlying skin is characteristically warm and red. Early in the disease, flecks of purulent material can be expressed from the salivary duct orifice. Intraorally the parotid papilla may be inflamed and pus may exude or be milked from the duct of the affected gland. Cervical lymphadenopathy usually develops.

Treatment usually starts with high dose of parenteral antibiotics active against penicillin resistant Staphylococcus.

Chronic Bacterial Sialadenitis

It is usually caused by *Streptococcus viridans*, *E. coli* or *Proteus*. As compared to acute parotitis, it can be seen in normal children or in adults.

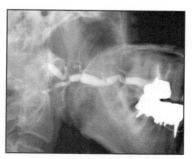

Fig. 17.10: Chronic sialadenitis. Sialogram shows marked dilation and strictures of the main ductal system. The parenchyma of the gland is poorly demonstrated (*Courtesy:* M Shizumu)

Recurrent form is most often due to duct obstruction, congenital stenosis, Sjögren's syndrome, or previous viral infection or allergy. It appears as a unilateral swelling at the angle of the jaw in a patient with the history of similar occurrence. Salivary flow is accompanied by flecks of purulent material. After several recurrences, fibrosis of the glandular parenchyma occurs, which leads to decreased salivary flow. The pain is usually minimal and antibiotic therapy resolves the infection within a week.

Sialograms show multiple ectasias and dilatation of the main excretory duct (Fig. 17.10).

AUTOIMMUNE DISORDERS

Sjögren's Syndrome

It is a chronic inflammatory disease that predominately affects salivary, lacrimal and other exocrine glands. It was first described by *Henrik Sjögren* in 1933. It predominately affects middle aged and elderly women.

It can be p*rimary Sjögren's syndrome (*sicca syndrome and it consists of dry eyes (xerophthalmia) and dry mouth (xerostomia), s*econdary Sjögren's syndrome* (dry eyes, dry mouth and collagen disorders usually rheumatoid arthritis or systemic lupus erythematous).

Xerostomia is a major complaint in most of the patients. There is difficulty in eating dry food, soreness or difficulty in controlling dentures. Pus may be emitted from the duct. Angular stomatitis and denture stomatitis also occur. Dry mouth may be accompanied by unilateral or bilateral enlargement of parotid gland, which occurs in about one third of the patients. Enlargement of submandibular gland may also occur. Clinically, the mouth may appear moist in early stages of Sjögren's syndrome but later, there may a lack of the usual pooling of saliva in the floor of the mouth and frothy saliva may form along the lines of contact with oral soft tissue. In advanced cases the mucosa is glazed, dry and tends to form fine wrinkles. The tongue typically develops a characteristic lobulated, usually red surface with partial or complete depapillation. There is also decrease in number of taste buds, which leads to an abnormal and impaired sense of taste.

General

The patient usually complains of dry eyes or continuous irritation in the eyes. Severe lacrimal gland involvement may lead to corneal ulceration as well as conjunctivitis. In patients with secondary Sjögren's syndrome, rheumatoid arthritis is typically long standing and clinically obvious. Patients may have small joint and ulnar deviation of fingers and rheumatoid nodules. This is accompanied by lack of secretion in the upper respiratory tract, may lead to pneumonia. Vaginal dryness may be also complained by some females.

Radiologically if the salivary flow rate is equivocal, sialography can be used to detect the damage. The most typical finding in Sjögren's syndrome is that of '*sialectasia*', which typically produces a '*snowstorm appearance*' as a result of leakage of contrast medium (Fig. 17.11). Atrophy of ductal tree may also be seen; emptying of the duct is also typically delayed (Fig. 17.12). In some cases it will show *'cherry blossom'* appearance of the obstructed ductal system. Salivary scintiscanning with technetium pertechnetate may be useful

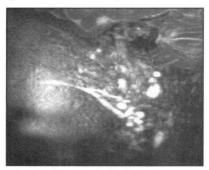

Fig. 17.11: MR sialography left parotid gland with Sjögren's syndrome, cavitary pattern. (Cases by *Courtesy:* of Tokyo Medical and Dental University, Japan)

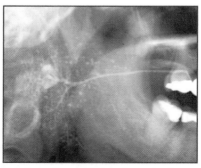

Fig. 17.12: Globular pattern with 1 to 2 mm in diameter collections of contrast material in periphery in Sjögren's syndrome

in demonstrating impaired salivary function in patients with Sjögren's syndrome. The changes correlate with, both, salivary flow rate and labial gland abnormalities.

Most of the patients are treated symptomatically.

Mikulicz's Disease or Benign Lymphoepithelial Lesion

It was first described by Mikulicz in 1888 as symmetric or bilateral, chronic, painless enlargement of lacrimal and salivary glands. It exhibits both inflammatory and neoplastic characteristics.

It can be *Mikulicz's disease proper* (lacrimal and salivary gland swelling only), *pseudo-leukemia* (lacrimal and salivary gland swelling plus lymphatic system involvement), *Leukemia* (lacrimal and salivary gland swelling plus hematopoietic involvement).

In some cases there is mild local discomfort, occasional pain and xerostomia. There is often diffuse, poorly outlined enlargement of salivary gland rather than formation of a discrete tumor nodule. There is history of alternating increases and decreases in the size of mass, from time to time. The duration of the tumor mass may be only a few months or many years.

Surgical excision and radiation can be given. Prognosis is good.

Tumors of Salivary Glands

It is important to note that neoplasms arise not only in major salivary glands, but also in minor salivary glands.

BENIGN TUMORS

Pleomorphic Adenoma

The term pleomorphic adenoma was suggested by Willis characterizing the unusual histological pattern of the lesion (pleomorphic or mixed appearance). It is a benign mixed tumor of the salivary gland. It is also called as *'iceberg tumor'*, *'endothelioma'*, *'branchioma'*, or *'enchondroma'*. It is most common of all the salivary gland tumor.

Small, painless, quiescent nodule which slowly begins to increase in size, sometimes intermittently. The tumor tends to be round or oval when it is small; as it grows bigger it becomes lobulated (Fig. 17.13). It may increase to cricket ball size or even more, weighing in pounds and in intraoral cases, not more than 1 to 2 cm in diameter. Its surface is smooth. Sometime it is bosselated and is occasionally crossed by deep furrows. No fixation, either to deeper tissues or overlying skin. It is firm and rubbery to feel. Sometimes

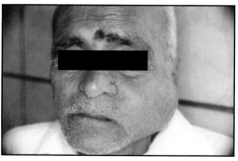

Fig. 17.13: Pleomorphic adenoma showing swelling in parotid region

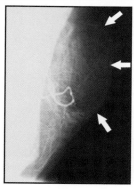

Fig. 17.14: Pleomorphic adenoma. Sialogram shows in the left parotid gland that some ducts are bent and displaced by the tumor; however, tumor itself (arrows) can not be seen ball in hand appearance

cystic degeneration may be seen. Sitography will produce ball in hand apperance (Fig. 17.14).

It is managed surgical excision.

Warthin's Tumor

It is also called as *'adenolymphoma'* and *'primary cystadenoma lymphomatosum'*.

The usual complaint is painless slow growing tumor over the angle of jaw. Involvement may be bilateral or may be multifocal. The tumor does not attain a large size and the usual size is 1-3 cm in diameter. It is spherical in shape. It is smooth and it is well circumscribed, movable. It classically feels doughy and compressible on palpation. It is firm on palpation and is clinically indistinguishable from other

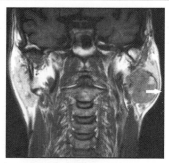

Fig. 17.15: Warthin's tumor: T1 weighted MR image shows round shaped mass with smooth, well-delineated contour in the lower pole of the left parotid gland. Signal intensity is higher than that of muscle

benign lesions of parotid gland. MRI image shows round shaped mass (Fig. 17.15).

Superficial parotidectomy and it seldom recurs after removal.

MALIGNANT TUMORS

Peripheral Mucoepidermoid Tumor

The term mucoepidermoid tumor was introduced in 1945 by Stewart, Foote and Becker.

It is of mainly two types, i.e. benign and malignant based upon clinical nature and histologic feature of the lesion.

It is usually not completely encapsulated and often contains cysts which may be filled with viscid mucoid material. The tumor of low grade malignancy usually appears as a slowly enlarging, painless mass, which stimulates pleomorphic adenoma. It has seldom exceed

5 cm in diameter (Figs 17.16 and 17.17). The tumor of high grade malignancy grows rapidly and does produce pain as an early symptom. It tends to infiltrate the surrounding tissues and in high percentage of cases it metastasizes to

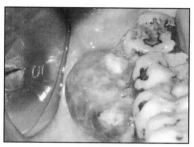

Fig. 17.16: Mucoepidermoid carcinoma showing ulcerated growth (*Courtesy:* Dr Abhishek Soni, Lecturer, Periodontology, VSPM Dental College and Research Centre, Nagpur, India)

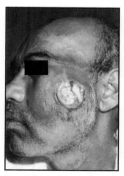

Fig. 17.17: Mucoepidermoid carcinoma present in the region of parotid region

the regional lymph nodes. Much more various findings such as lacrimation, trismus, nasal discharge, blood tinged saliva and facial nerve paralysis are seen in high grade malignant lesions.

Surgical excision followed by radiotherapy is recommended for intermediate grade tumors and high grade tumors. Low grade tumors can be managed by surgery alone.

Adenoid Cystic Carcinoma (Fig 17.18)

It is also called as *'cylindroma'*, *'adenocystic carcinoma'* and *'baseloid mixed tumor'*.

The most common initial symptom is presence of mass followed by local pain, facial nerve paralysis in case of parotid tumor and tenderness. Some of the lesions exhibit surface ulceration. Other findings include nasal obstruction, proptosis, sinusitis, ear infection, epistaxis, signs of cranial nerve involvement and visual disturbances.

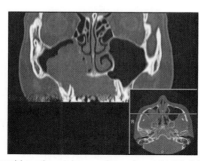

Fig. 17.18: Adenoid cystic carcinoma shows (on right 5 kg) bone destruction and absorption of the dental root. Some fine calcification can also be seen in the tumor

Surgical and in some cases it is accompanied by X-ray radiation.

Malignant Pleomorphic Adenoma (Fig. 17.19)

It is also called as *'malignant mixed tumor'*. It is uncertain that these tumors represent the previously benign lesions which have undergone transformation into malignant form or are malignant lesion right from the onset.

The tumors are usually larger than benign ones. There is often fixation of the tumor to underlying structures as well as to overlying skin or mucosa. Pain is more frequently

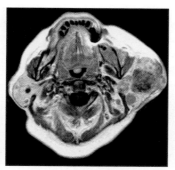

Fig. 17.19: Malignant pleomorphic adenoma presented as growth on left side

a feature of malignant, than the benign pleomorphic adenoma.

These neoplasms exhibit a high recurrence rate after surgical removal as well as a high incidence of regional lymph node involvement.

Disorders of Maxillary Sinus

Paranasal sinuses are the air filled spaces present with some bone around the nasal cavities (Fig. 18.1). The sinuses are frontal, maxillary, sphenoidal and ethmoidal. Because of the close proximity of the maxillary teeth with the maxillary sinuses, they are the most important paranasal sinus from dental point of view. They are the largest air filled sinuses surrounding the nose.

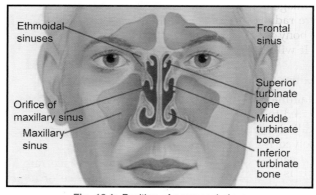

Fig. 18.1: Position of paranasal sinus

INFLAMMATORY

They are caused by chemical irritation, introduction of foreign body, facial trauma, etc.

Mucositis

It is the name given when there is thickened mucous membrane of maxillary sinus. Normally, mucous membrane of maxillary sinus is about 1 mm in thickness. When the lining mucosa becomes inflamed from either infection or an allergic process, it may increase in thickness by about 10 to 15 times. This inflammation is called as mucositis.

It is caused by dental inflammatory lesion such as periodontal disease or periapical disease may cause localized mucositis.

It is usually asymptomatic and it is discovered on routine radiograph.

Image is detected on a radiograph as a band, noticeable more radiopaque than the air filled sinus and paralleling the bony wall of the sinus (Fig. 18.2).

It will disappear after removing the cause.

Maxillary Sinusitis

Inflammation of the mucosa of the paranasal sinuses is referred to as sinusitis. When maxillary sinus is involved it is called as maxillary sinusitis. When all the sinuses are involved it is called a pansinusitis.

It can be acute, subacute and chronic types.

It is caused by periapical infection from the teeth,

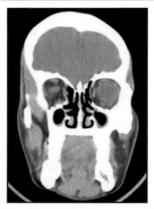

Fig. 18.2: CT coronal section showing fine mucosal thickening, involving medial and lateral wall along with the floor of the Maxillary Sinus bilaterally

oroantral fistula, periodontitis, and traumatic, dental material in the antrum, implant, and infected dental cyst. It can be caused by mechanical obstruction of ostium, common cold, allergic rhinitis, deviated nasal septum, presence of nasal polyp and prolonged nasotracheal intubation.

Acute maxillary sinusitis - The main symptom is severe pain which is constant and localized. Pain may be felt in the area of eyeball, cheek and frontal region. Pain may be exacerbated by stooping or lowering the head. Post nasal drip causing irritation, stuffiness and nasal discharge. Pain in the teeth may be referred to the premolars and molars on the affected side. Teeth in the involved side become sore and painful. Nasal discharge is watery in the beginning but later becomes mucopurulent. In cases of sinusitis from infected teeth, the discharge has a foul odor. Tenderness to pressure or swelling over the involved sinus. Intraorally, there may be a mucobuccal swelling, reddening and pain near the sinus region.

Subacute - It is an interim stage between acute and chronic sinusitis. It is devoid of symptoms associated with acute congestion such as pain and generalized toxemia. Discharge is usually purulent and associated with a nasal voice and stuffiness. Soreness of throat is common.

Chronic - It develops as a result of neglected and overlooked dental focus of infection. The lining becomes thicker and irregular. General symptoms of chronic sinusitis include sense of tiredness, low grade fever and feeling of being unwell. Stuffy sensation over the affected side of the face. Nasal obstruction, nasal discharge and headache are the related symptoms.

Radiologically four patterns are seen, i.e. localized thickening at the base of the sinus, roughly generalized thickening of mucoperiosteum around the entire wall of the sinus, complete filling of the sinus except in the region of the osteum on the medial wall and complete filling of the sinus (Figs 18.3 and 18.4). Mucosal thickening may be uniform or polypoid. Chronic sinusitis may result in persistent opacification of the sinus and sclerosis or thickening of surrounding bone.

It is managed by antibiotic, analgesic and anti-inflammatory drugs, nasal decongestant, stem inhalation, antral lavage, and antrostomy.

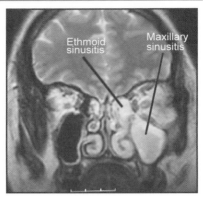

Fig. 18.3: CT scan of maxillary and ethmoid sinusitis

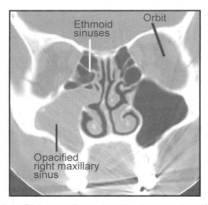

Fig. 18.4: Right maxillary sinusitis showing opacification

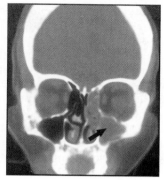

Fig. 18.5: Sinusitis occurring due to Aspergillus infection (arrow)

Empyema

If sinus ostium remains blocked by thickened inflamed mucosa or other pathological conditions, an empyema is possible, which is 'cavity filled with pus'.

Radiographically sinus will appear completely opaque (Fig. 18.5). Decalcification of surrounding bony walls and haziness of trabecular bone next to the sinus wall is seen. It may extend into the adjacent bone with development of osteomyelitis.

CYST

Benign Mucosal Cyst of Maxillary Antrum

It is also called as, 'retention cyst', 'pseudocyst', 'lymphangiectatic cyst', 'false cyst', 'benign mucosal antral cyst', 'serous non-secretory retention pseudocyst', 'mesothelial cyst' and 'intramural cyst'.

The mucus secretory retention cyst results from obstruction of the duct of seromucinous gland in lamina propria of the sinus lining caused by infection and allergy.

The serous, non-secretory retention cyst arises as a result of cystic degeneration within an inflamed thickened sinus lining or in mucosal polyp space.

There may be localized dull pain in the antral region, or fullness and numbness of the cheek. If it is a completely filled sinus, it will prolapse through the ostium and cause obstruction and post nasal drip. There may be pain in the teeth and face over or near the sinus. There may be stuffiness, fullness, and headache, symptoms of cold and numbness of upper lip. Retention pseudocyst may enlarge and fills the sinus cavity completely, it frequently rupture as a result of abrupt pressure change caused by sneezing or blowing the nose.

Radiologically present as homogenous mass that is more radiopaque than the surrounding sinus cavity. It is found projecting from the floor of the sinus, although some may form on the lateral walls (Fig. 18.6). The cyst appears as a spherical, ovoid or dome shaped radio-opacity. It has a smooth and uniform outline. They may have a narrow or broad base. They vary in size from minute to very large and may occasionally occupy the entire maxillary sinus.

Large cysts should be removed through Caldwell-luc operation.

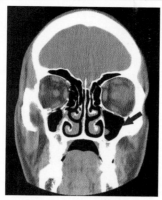

Fig. 18.6: CT coronal section showing fine mucosal thickening in Rt. Max. Sinus and mucous retention cyst (Arrow mark) involving Lt. Maxillary Sinus

Mucocele

It is an expanding destructive lesion that begins with the development of mucus retention cyst in a blocked ostium. If mucocele becomes infected, it is called as pyocele or mucopyocele.

It may exert pressure on the superior alveolar nerve in the resorbing sinus wall and cause radiating pain. Sensation of fullness in the cheek may be accompanied by swelling over the anteroinferior aspect of the antrum the area where the wall is thinnest. If the cyst expands inferiorly, it may cause loosening of the posterior teeth in that area. If it

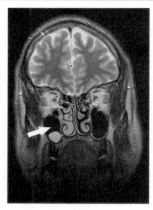

Fig. 18.7: MRI T2 coronal section image showing well marginated hyper intense area in the floor of the Rt. Max. Sinus (Arrow mark) suggestive of solitary polyp

expands medially, lateral wall of the nasal cavity is deformed and nasal air way is obstructed. If expands towards the orbit it may cause diplopia and proptosis (protrusion of the globe of the eye).

Radiographically there is opacification of sinus. The shape of the sinus is changed into a more circular shape as the mucocele grows (Fig. 18.7). The shape of sinuses changes with bony expansion. Erosion of septa and the bony wall may occur. Borders of the expanding sinus become sclerotic. Teeth may be displaced or resorbed.

Surgical removal by the Caldwell Luc operation.

MALIGNANT TUMOR

Squamous Cell Carcinoma

It originates from metaplastic epithelium of the sinus mucous membrane lining.

It is caused by sinusitis, snuff and smoke. There is facial pain, swelling, nasal obstruction and lymphadenopathy. Medial wall involvement leads to nasal obstruction, discharge, bleeding and pain. Epiphora will result if the lacrimal sac or nasolacrimal duct is obstructed. Involvement of the floor of the sinus leads to expansion of the alveolus, unexplained pain, numbness of teeth, loose teeth and swelling of the palate or alveolar ridge and malfitting dentures. It may erode the floor and penetrate the oral cavity (Fig. 18.8).

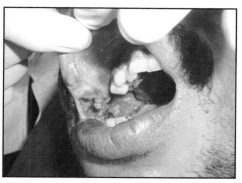

Fig. 18.8: Maxillary sinus malignancy, presented as a growth inside the oral cavity

Lateral wall involvement leads to facial and vestibular swelling (Fig. 18.9), pain and hyperesthesia of maxillary teeth. Roof involvement leads to diplopia, proptosis and pain over the cheek and upper teeth. Posterior wall involvement leads to painful trismus, obstruction of eustachian tube causing stuffy ear, referred pain and hyperesthesia over the distribution of second and third division of trigeminal nerve. It may involve infraorbital nerve and produces paresthesia of the cheek or erodes blood vessels giving rise to epistaxis.

Radiologically there is non-specific well defined round soft tissue opacity within the antrum. Variable destruction of the bony antral wall (Fig. 18.10). Loss of fine linear outline of the lateral wall is a particularly sensitive sign of bone

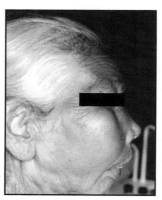

Fig. 18.9: Maxillary antrum malignancy showing extraoral swelling in sinus area

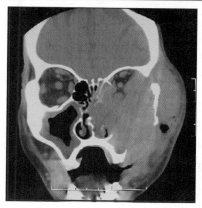

Fig. 18.10: Malignancy on right maxillary sinus showing destruction upto the orbits

destruction. In larger lesion destructive outline of the sinus destroying bone and causing irregular bony radiolucency with erosion of the medial wall (Fig. 18.11). There may be destruction of the floor and anterior or posterior walls.

Occasional resorption and displacement of the teeth. There may be bone destruction around the teeth or irregular widening of the periodontal ligament space. Advanced cases involve destruction of the zygomatic arch. On the tomography, there is destruction of the surrounding hard and soft tissue.

It is managed by local intra-arterial infusion of cytotoxic drugs, radiotherapy and chemotherapy. After surgery sophisticated prosthesis should be constructed.

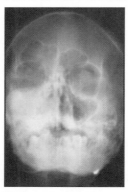

Fig. 18.11: Maxillary sinus malignancy on left side showing complete radiopacification of sinus

TRAUMATIC INJURIES TO THE PARANASAL SINUSES

Root in Antrum

In maxillary posterior teeth, it is possible that fractured root tip may be forced in to the maxillary sinus either while extraction or while removing the root tip. If root tip is in the socket and superimposed over the sinus then lamina dura will be intact and it is in maxillary sinus lamina dura will be lost. When root tip is in the sinus and trapped under mucoperiosteum then it will be fixed and it may cause movement when it perforates the sinus. Removal of the root tip can be done through the tooth socket or though the canine fossa by Caldwell-Luc approach.

Oroantral Fistula

It is a pathological pathway connecting oral cavity and maxillary sinus. If there is no pathological lining present it is called as oroantral opening which is seen after tooth extraction.

It causes inappropriate or incorrect use of elevators during root or tooth removal. Forceps extraction of a solitary isolated premolar or molar in an edentulous part of the arch is also prone to cause disruption of the sinus floor, blind instrumentation without adequate surgical exposure, in cases of removal of cysts and benign tumors in upper posterior region, massive trauma to the middle third of the facial skeleton, malignant tumors of the maxillary sinus.

Oroantral opening can be seen immediately after extraction of the tooth (Fig. 18.12). Immediate symptoms includes passage of fluid from oral cavity into the nose.

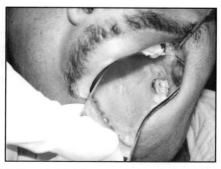

Fig. 18.12: Oroantral fistula presented as an opening intraorally

Inability to blow out cheek and smoke cigarettes. Unilateral epistaxis, due to blood in the maxillary sinus escaping through the nasal ostium. There may be escape of air from the mouth into the nose and an alteration in vocal resonance. Delayed symptoms includes foul, sweetish fetid or salty taste in mouth, facial pain or headache which is of throbbing nature and is exacerbated by movement of the head. Unilateral nasal discharge accompanied by sensation of nasal obstruction or nocturnal coughing resulting from draining of exudate into pharynx.

Radiograph will show break in continuity of maxillary sinus (Fig. 18.13). In some cases there is disalignment of a

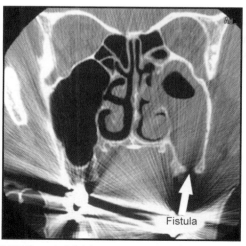

Fig. 18.13: Oroantral fistula seen as an opening on the CT scan

small portion of the cortical layer of bone. There are also characteristic features of acute or chronic sinusitis due to ingress of bacteria.Evidence of displaced root or tooth and second view of the antrum with the head in a different position may be required to ascertain the exact location of the displaced object.

It is managed by antibiotic therapy for 1 week. Most commonly given antibiotics is amoxicillin. Decongestants are given for 1 week.

CALCIFICATION

Antroliths

These are calcified masses found in the maxillary sinus. It is defined as a complete or partial calcific encrustation of an antral foreign body, either endogenous or exogenous which serves as nidus. There is calcification of masses of

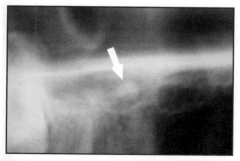

Fig. 18.14: Periapical radiograph showing antrolith (arrow) (*Courtesy:* Dr Enzio Rovigatti)

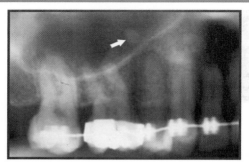

Fig. 18.15: Antrolith in right maxillary sinus
(*Courtesy:* Dr Enzio Rovigatti)

stagnant mucus in site of previous inflammation, root fragments or bone chips or foreign body.

It is caused by endogenous nidus in usually root tip or may be simply fragment of soft tissue, bone, blood or mucus. Exogenous nidi are consisting of snuff or paper.

It is usually asymptomatic. But if they continue to grow the patient may complain of bloodstained nasal discharge, nasal obstruction or facial pain.

Radiologically they may have a homogeneous or heterogeneous density. There is alternating layer of radiolucency and radiopacity in the form of lamination. Outline may be ragged or smooth. Shape may be round, oval or irregular and it is attached to the wall of the sinus (Figs 18.14 and 18.15).

Removal of antroliths can be done if it is symptomatic.

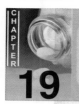
Trauma of Teeth and Facial Structure

TRAUMATIC INJURY TO SOFT TISSUE

Traumatic Erythematous Macule and Erosion

It is induced by low grade, usually chronic, physical insult.

Size of red zone corresponds too closely to size of traumatic agent (19.1). Margins are not sharply defined. Mild to considerable pain and it regresses after the cause is removed. It may blanch when digital pressure is used.

Mechanical irritant is identified and removed.

Electrical Burns

It occurs more frequently at the commissure region of the lips. It occurs in when the child chews electrical cords, breaks the insulation and contacts the bare wire or sucks on the socket ends of an extension cords. The tissue is burnt by thermal changes at the entrance and exit sites of the current.

The clinical appearance of the burn is a gray white tissue surrounded by narrow rim of erythema. The center of the lesion may be depressed and margins are raised. As there is destruction of neural tissue the lesions are usually painless

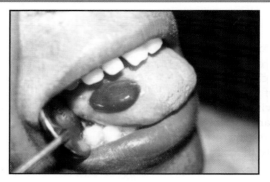

Fig. 19.1: Traumatic hematoma occurring on
dorsal surface of the tongue

and some sensory and motor loss may result in the
surrounding tissues. Tissue begins to swell within the few
hours of injury, the margin of wound become irregular and
the lips protrude and control of saliva is diminished.
Following sloughing, irregular ulceration can occur. The
result of electrical trauma is characterized by coagulation
of protein, liquefaction of fat and vaporization of tissue
fluids.

Traumatic Injury to Teeth

There are various causes of traumatic injuries to teeth like
falls, collisions, sporting activities, domestic violence,
automobile accident and assault.

FRACTURE OF TEETH

Dental Crown Fracture

Anterior teeth are commonly involved. It may be caused by fall, accident and blows from foreign bodies.

It can be crack (fracture involve only enamel without loss of enamel substance), uncomplicated fracture (fracture involving enamel or enamel and dentin with loss of tooth substance without pulpal involvement) and complicated fracture (fracture that extends through enamel, dentin and pulp with loss of tooth substance).

Cracks: It can be seen in indirect light (directing the beam along the long axis of tooth).

Uncomplicated fracture: It does not involve dentin and is usually found on mesial or distal corner of maxillary central incisors. Dentin involvement is identified by contrast of color between it and peripheral layer of enamel. Exposed dentin is very sensitive to chemical, thermal and mechanical stimulation (Fig. 19.2).

Complicated fractures: There is bleeding from exposed pulp or at least drop of blood oozes from the pinpoint exposure. Exposed pulp will be sensitive to most forms of stimulation.

Radiologically it will show size and position of pulp chamber, location and extent of exposure and stage of root development (Fig. 19.3).

It is managed by pulp capping, pulpotomy and pulpectomy can be done.

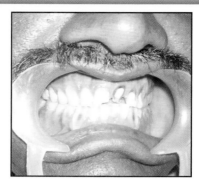

Fig. 19.2: Incisal fracture of upper right central
incisors due to traumatic occlusion

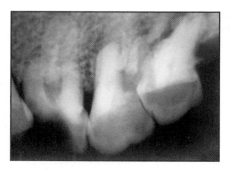

Fig. 19.3: Fracture of crown of first molar
may occur due to carious process

Dental Root Fracture

Coronal fragment is displaced lingually and is slightly extruded. If fracture line is close to the apex then tooth will be more stable. If only movement of crown is detected, root fracture is likely.

Radiologically if the X-ray beam is projected parallel with the plane of the root, sharp radiolucent line between the fragments can be seen (Fig. 19.4). If the X-ray beam is not parallel, it will look as poorly defined gray shadow. Fracture line may be transverse or oblique.

Teeth mainly restored to their proper position and securely immobilized.

Crown/root Fracture

Such fracture is likely to be intra and extra alveolar. They are a result of direct trauma. There is pain during mastication. Tooth is sensitive to occlusal force.

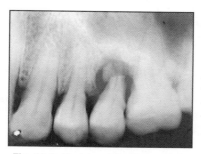

Fig. 19.4: Dental root fracture seen in association with second premolar

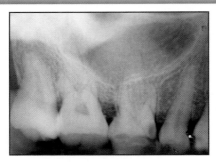

Fig. 19.5: Fracture cusp of crowing which also extending into the root of first molar occur due to occlusal trauma

Most crown-root fractures are perpendicular to the direction of the beam (Fig. 19.5).

Removal of coronal fragment: If 3 to 4 mm of root is remaining, extraction is indicated.

Vertical Root Fracture

It is also called as 'cracked tooth syndrome'. It runs length wise from crown towards apex of tooth.

It is caused by iatrogenic cause, endodontically treated tooth and traumatic occlusion.

Dull pain of long duration which may vary from non existent to mild.

Radiologically if central X-ray lies in the plane of the fracture, it may be visible as a radiolucent line.

Traumatic Injury to Facial Bone

When patient is subjected to injury, there is chance that jaws may be fractured. Even in some cases minor trauma may result in bone damage.

Mandibular Fractures

Fracture of mandible occurs more frequently than any other fracture of the facial skeleton. The most common facial fracture is mandible (61%), followed by maxilla (46%), the zygoma (27%) and the nasal bones (19%).

It is caused by road traffic accidents, assault, falls, industrial trauma and sport injury.

It can be simple (closed linear fracture of the condyle, coronoid, ramus and edentulous body of the mandible) Greenstick (occur in children), compound (tooth bearing portions of the mandible are nearly always compound into the mouth via the periodontal membrane) comminuted (direct violence to mandible from penetrating sharp objects and missiles) and pathological (when fractures result from minimum trauma to mandible which is already weakened by pathological conditions).

Dentoalveolar Fractures

These are defined as those in which avulsion, subluxation or fracture of teeth occur in relation with fracture of the alveolus. It may occur alone or in combination with other mandibular fractures.

There is full thickness wound of the lower lip or ragged laceration on its inner aspect caused by impaction against the lower anterior teeth. There may be local bruising and portions of teeth or foreign bodies may get lodged in soft tissue of lip. There may be fracture of crown and root portion of teeth. There may be gross comminution of alveolus.

Coronoid Fracture

It is rare. Usually results from reflex contracture of the powerful anterior fibers of temporalis muscle during operation on large cyst of ramus.

If the tip of the coronoid process is ditched, the fragment is pulled upwards towards the infratemporal fossa by the temporalis muscle. There may be tenderness over the anterior part of the ramus and hematoma. Painful limitation of movement, especially on protrusion of mandible may be found.

Fracture of Ramus

Single fracture: It is low condylar fracture with both the coronoid and condylar process on the upper fragment.

Comminuted fracture: It results from direct violence to the side of face.

Swelling and ecchymosis is usually noted extra and intraorally. There is tenderness over the ramus and movements produce pain over the same area. Severe trismus may be present.

Fractures at Angle of Mandible (Figs 19.6 and 19.7)

There is swelling at the angle externally and there is obvious deformity. Anesthesia or paresthesia of the lower lip may be present on the side of fracture.

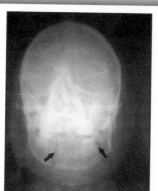

Fig. 19.6: Horizontally unfavorable fracture of the angle of mandible and parasymphysial fracture involving the teeth in fracture line

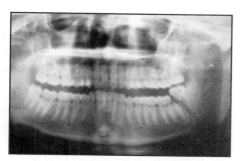

Fig. 19.7: Fracture line seen at angle of mandible on left side going through the root of third molar also

Intraorally, there is step deformity which can be seen behind the last molar. The occlusion is often deranged with tenderness at angle of mandible. Movement and crepitus at the fracture site can be felt, if the ramus is steadied between finger and thumb and the body of the mandible moved gently with the other hand. Movement of mandible is painful and trismus is usually present to some degree.

Fracture of Mandibular Body (Fig. 19.8)

It can be unfavorable (the fracture line in the body of mandible starts posteriorly and inferiorly such that the masseter and internal pterygoid muscles pull the ramus segment away from the body of mandible, the fracture is said to be unfavorable) or favorable (in favorable fractures, muscle action reduces the fracture).

Fracture of the mandibular body on one side is frequently accompanied by fracture of condyle on the opposite side. There may be unilateral pain present inspite of bilateral

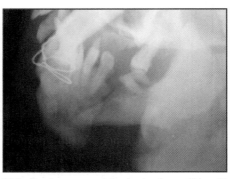

Fig 19.8: Fracture seen at the body of mandible with displacement of segment of the jaw

fracture. Contusion and wounds on skin. Discrepancy in occlusal plane.

Ecchymosis in the floor of mouth. In some cases, inferior dental artery may be torn giving rise to severe intraoral hemorrhage. Since the tongue is attached to the anterior fragment, it is possible in the recumbent position for the tongue to fall back and obstruct the glottis with fatal results.

Fractures of Symphysis and Parasymphysis (Figs 19.9 to 19.11)

These fractures are usually associated with fracture of one or both condyles. The presence of bony tenderness and a small lingual hematoma may be the only physical signs.

As such, fracture is a result of direct violence there is frequently associated soft tissue injury of the chin and lower

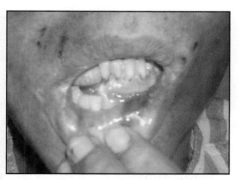

Fig. 19.9: Step deformity seen in the fracture of mandible in the symphysis region

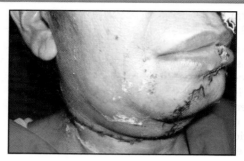

Fig. 19.10: Fracture in symphysis region. Photographs taken after suturing is done

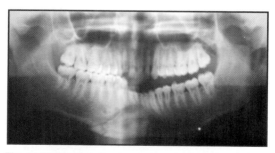

Fig. 19.11: Fracture line in parasymphysis and symphysis region also showing fracture condyle on left side

lip. In some cases, there is detachment of the genioglossus muscle which may contribute to the loss of tongue control and obstruction of airway.

Radiographic Features of Mandibular Fracture (Figs 19.12 to 19.14)

There is sharp, well defined radiolucent line separating the fracture segments of bone. Fracture through the buccal and lingual cortical plates may produce two radiolucent lines. If there is displacement, cortical discontinuity or step will be evident. Irregularity in occlusal plane. Bilateral fracture of body of mandible is sometimes followed by downward angulation of the anterior fragment. Sometimes, it will overlap each other giving rise to radiopaque line at site.

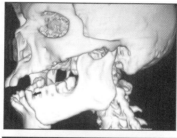

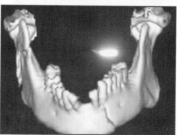

Fig. 19.12: 3D CT image of mandibular fracture at symphysis region (*Courtesy:* Dr Amit Parate, Lecturer, GDCH, Nagpur, India)

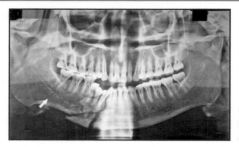

Fig. 19.13: Displacement of the fractured segment resulting in step deformity at the lower border

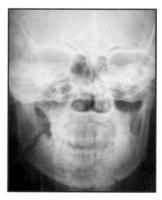

Fig. 19.14: Multiple fractures seen in mandible due to major trauma

All fracture of mandible are managed by reduction, immobilization of fractured bone.

MIDDLE THIRD FRACTURES

Alveolar Ridge

It involves lingual wall of alveolar ridge. Anterior alveolar fractures are most common. Labial plate is more prone to fracture than palatal plate. Fracture line is most often horizontal. Marked malocclusion along with displacement and mobility (Figs 19.15 and 19.16). The detached bone may include the floor of maxillary sinus; which is indicated by discharge from the nose on the involved side. Ecchymosis of buccal vestibule can also occur.

Radiologically damage to roots of the adjacent teeth is common with fracture of alveolus, fracture of alveolar process is well delineated and posterior palate fracture is best demonstrated on occlusal radiograph.

It is managed by splinting of teeth and anchoring the tooth.

Mid Facial Fracture

It may involve the frontal, nasal, lacrimal, zygoma, ethmoidal and sphenoid bones. They are classified by Rene Le Fort.

Le Fort I

It is also called as 'low level fracture'. It is a horizontal fracture above the level of nasal floor. It results in maxillary tooth bearing fragment being detached from the midface.

Fracture line passes above the teeth, from lateral margin of the anterior nasal aperture below the zygomatic buttress through the maxillary sinus, tuberosity and to the inferior portion of the pterygoid palate.

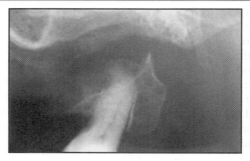

Fig. 19.15: Fracture of maxillary tuberosity with
displacement of fracture segment

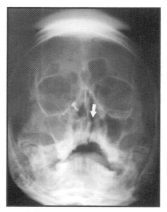

Fig. 19.16: Transverse fracture of maxilla in water view

In recent injury there may be slight swelling of upper lip. Some fractures are so mobile that the patient has to keep the mouth slightly open to accommodate the increased vertical dimension of bite. Paresthesia over the distribution of infra-orbital nerve. Pain over nose and face.

Occlusion is disturbed and variable amount of mobility may be found in the tooth bearing segment of maxilla. In impacted type of fracture there may be damage to cusps of individual teeth caused by impaction of the mandibular teeth against them. Percussion of upper teeth results in a distinctive 'cracked pot' sound. The complete Le Fort fracture is often associated with a split in the palate.

Radiologically identified on PA, lateral skull and Water's projection (Fig. 19.17). Both maxillary sinuses are cloudy

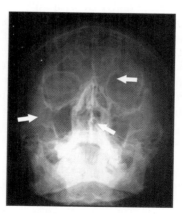

Fig 19.17: Waters view showing Le-Fort I fracture with fracture of zygomatic bone

and may show air filled level. Lateral view shows slight posterior displacement of fragment.

It is managed by intermaxillary fixation.

Le Fort II

It is also called as 'pyramidal or subzygomatic fracture'. There is a pyramidal appearance of fracture in PA skull view.

This fracture line runs from the thin middle area of the nasal bone, on either side, crossing the frontal processes of the maxilla into the medial wall of each orbit. Within each orbit, the fracture line crosses the lacrimal bone behind lacrimal sac, before turning forward to cross the infraorbital margin slightly medial to or through infraorbital foramen. The fracture now extends downwards and backwards across the lateral wall of the antrum, below the zygomaticomaxillary suture and divides the pterygoid laminae about halfway up.

There is massive edema that cause marked swelling of the middle third of face giving rise to 'moon face' appearance. There is bilateral circumorbital ecchymosis, subconjunctival ecchymosis and periorbital hematoma (Fig. 19.18). There may be diplopia and ocular movements may be limited. There may be lengthening of the nose. There may be bleeding from the nose. As the fracture line passes across the inferior orbital rim, there may be injury to the infraorbital nerve resulting in anesthesia or paresthesia of cheek. There is step deformity at infraorbital margin.

Radiologically it will reveal fracture of the nasal bone and both, frontal processes of maxilla and infra-orbital rims

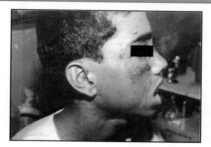

Fig. 19.18: Le Fort II fracture showing
swelling in the maxillary region

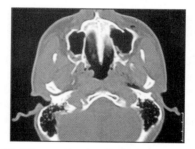

Fig. 19.19: CT scan showing the fracture at anterior and
posterior wall of maxillary sinus

on both sides or separation of zygomatic sutures on both
sides. Deformities and discontinuation of lateral walls of
both sides of maxillary sinus (Fig. 19.19). Thickening of the
lining mucosa and clouding of maxillary sinus.

It is managed by reduction followed by intermaxillary
fixation.

Le Fort III

It is also called as 'high transverse or suprazygomatic fracture'. It completely separates the middle third of the facial skeleton from the cranium.

Fracture line runs from near the frontonasal suture transversely backwards, parallel with the base of the skull and involves the full depth of the ethmoid bone, including cribriform plate. Within the orbit, the fracture passes below the optic foramen into the posterior limit of the inferior orbital fissure. From the base of the inferior orbital fissure, the fracture line extends in two directions: backwards across the pterygomaxillary fissure, to fracture the roots of the pterygoid laminae and laterally across the lateral wall of the orbit separating the zygomatic bone from the frontal bone.

Superficially it appears similar to Le Fort II but injury is much more severe. It is very unusual to find Le Fort III fracture occurring in isolation. It is more extensive and massive. There is tenderness and often separation at the frontozygomatic sutures. There may be mobility of whole of the facial skeleton as a single block. Nose often blocked with blood clot. Cerebrospinal fluid rhinorrhea will be profuse as compared to Le Fort II. There is bleeding into periorbital tissues. There is separation of both frontozygomatic sutures which produces lengthening of face. The entire occlusal plane may drop producing anterior open bite. There is gagging of occlusion in the molar area.

Radiologically hazy due to soft tissue swelling. Separation of sutures i.e. of nasofrontal process, maxillofrontal, zygomaticofrontal and zygomaticotemporal. Nasal bone, frontal process of maxilla, both orbital floors and pterygoid plate show radiolucent lines and discontinuity. Ethmoidal and sphenoid sinuses are cloudy.

It is managed by external immobilization.

Zygomatic Fracture

It can be of zygomatic arch and zygomatic complex.

Zygomatic arch: Arch may fracture at its center resulting in a V-shaped medial displacement (Fig. 19.20). Fracture of zygomatic arch tends to impinge on the coronoid process and so extreme interference with the mandibular movement may be found. There is depression over the zygomatic arch.

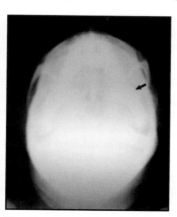

Fig. 19.20: Zygomatic arch fracture

Zygomatic complex: Tenderness is noted at fracture line. Step defect may be palpated in the zygomaticofrontal area and along the infraorbital rim. When the zygomatic bone is fractured near the zygomaticofrontal, zygomaticotemporal and zygomaticomaxillary sutures, it is most often displaced inwards to a greater or lesser extent. There may be minimum displacement or an obviously unsightly flattening of one cheek bone. Diplopia, enophthalmos, proptosis, dilating pupil, ophthalmoplegia and decreasing visual acuity. Blindness may follow in the absence of decompression and is caused by ischemia of a critical zone of optic nerve following occlusion or spasm of the short posterior ciliary arteries. Circumorbital ecchymosis occurs in most cases of zygomatic fracture. Fractures which involve the orbital wall tend to be accompanied by subconjunctival hemorrhage (Figs 19.21 and 19.22). Limitation of mandibular movements occurs if the displaced zygomatic bone impinges on the coronoid process.

Radiologically water's view will provide an image of the entire zygoma and maxillary sinus. Radiographs will show haziness caused by attending edema of the face. Separation or fracture of frontozygomatic suture. As the zygomatic bone is displaced into maxillary sinus in the region of the zygomaticomaxillary suture (Fig. 19.23), the outer wall of the antrum is comminuted and the antrum fills with the blood. On radiograph, it is seen as opacity.

Reduction and fixation can be done.

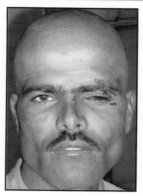

Fig. 19.21: Subconjunctival hemorrhage seen in zygomatico-maxillary complex fracture

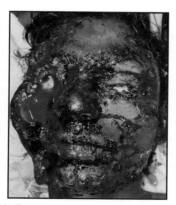

Fig 19.22: Extensive soft tissue injury associated with fracture of zygomaticomaxillary complex

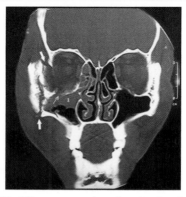

Fig. 19.23: CT scan coronal section showing the lateral displacement of fractured zygomatic bone fragment

Green Stick Fracture

It occurs in young people. Rare in maxilla and mandible. Radiologically, there is sharp angulation present at the site of fracture.

There may be one or more linear dark streaks running some distance along the length of the bones from each side of the angulation. Small spicules of bone may be seen standing away from the surface, which had been stripped away at the time of fracture.

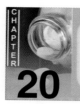
Soft Tissue Calcification

DYSTROPHIC CALCIFICATION

General Dystrophic Calcification of the Oral Region

When calcium salt precipitate into primary site of chronic inflammation, dead and dying tissue, it is called as dystrophic calcification. It is associated with high local concentration of phosphatase, as in normal bone calcification and with anoxic conditions within the devitalized tissue.

It is most frequent form of pathologic calcification and found in a wide variety of tissues like areas of tuberculosis, necrosis, and blood vessels in arteriosclerosis, scars and areas of fatty degeneration. In oral cavity, area of dystrophic degeneration is found in the gingiva, tongue or cheek. It is asymptomatic. Overlying tissue is enlarged and ulcerated and solid mass of calcium salt palpable.

Radiologically it appears as fine grains of radiopacities which are sparse and diffuse. It may be single or multiple and rarely exceed 0.5 cm in diameter. Outline is irregular or indistinct.

Calcified Lymph Nodes

These are types of dystrophic calcification that occurs in lymph nodes following chronic infections. Patient may recall a severe infection that could explain degeneration of lymphoid tissues.

It is usually asymptomatic. It may be single or multiple or some times chain of nodes. They are hard, round or oblong masses. Outline is well contoured and well defined. They are mobile during palpation.

Radiologically it is most commonly seen behind or below the angle of the mandible. In rare cases calcified node is found posterior to the ramus. It is opaque and well defined. In some cases radiodensity is variable showing both opaque and radiolucent appearance. It may have laminated appearance. Sometimes irregular heterogeneous opaque masses are seen which appear to resemble a *mass of coral*. Radiopacity often exhibits a patchy pattern with a reticular arrangement of radiolucent lines or gaps. Well defined and usually irregular, occasionally having a lobulated appearance similar to outer shape of cauliflower (Fig. 20.1).

Dystrophic Calcification in the Tonsil

It is also called as *'tonsillar calculi'*, *'tonsil concretions'*, and *'tonsilloliths'*. The mechanism is similar to that of calcified lymph nodes.

Small calcification produce no symptoms but larger calcification can produce pain, swelling and dysphagia.

Radiologically it can produce *'speckled'* appearances of multiple radiopaque superimposed bilaterally on the images

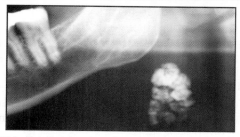

Fig. 20.1: Calcified lymph nodes, cervical lymph nodes that is cauliflower shaped and chainlike (*Courtesy:* Dr Enzio Rovigatti)

of the mandibular rami in a panoramic radiograph. It appears more radiopaque than the cancellous bone and same as cortical bone.

Cysticercosis

When eggs or gravid proglottids from *Taenia solium* (pork tapeworm) are ingested by human, their covering is digested in stomach and larval form (Cysticercus cellulosae) of the parasite is hatched. Larvae penetrate the mucosa, enter the blood vessels and lymphatics and are distributed in the tissue all over the body. After the larva die, the larval spaces are replaced with fibrous connective tissue, which may become calcified.

Mild cases are completely asymptomatic. In severe cases there is mild to severe GIT upset with epigastric pain, severe nausea and vomiting. Palpable firm mass upto 1 cm in diameter.

Radiologically the margins are well defined. The shape is elongated, elliptical or ovoid. It is homogenous and radiopaque.

Medical management by the physician.

Calcified Blood Vessels

Arterial wall may calcify in all forms of arteriosclerosis with deposition of calcium salts within the medial coat of the vessels.

It is sequelae of inflammatory process affecting the wall. It is also found in Sturge-Weber syndrome.

Usually no clinical sign or symptoms develop.

Radiologically, calcific deposits on wall of artery will outline the image of the artery. A pair of thin opaque lines that may have either a straight course or a tortuous path (Fig. 20.2). They may appear as amorphous or punctuate calcifications. The calcified wall appear as radiopaque circle.

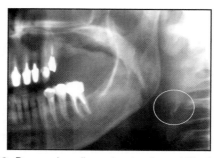

Fig. 20.2: Panoramic radiographs showing calcification in the carotid artery (*Courtesy:* Dr Fábio de Lima Cravo)

Idiopathic Calcification

The deposition of calcium in normal tissue despite normal serum calcium and phosphate level is referred to as 'idiopathic calcification'.

Phleboliths

These are thought to be formed in older thrombi in veins or hemangiomas with slow blood flow. The thrombus organizes into granulation tissue and occasionally mineralizes with the deposition of calcium phosphate and calcium carbonate.

The involved soft tissue may be swollen or discolored by the presence of veins or a soft tissue hemangioma. Applying pressure to the involved tissue should cause a blanching or change in color if the lesion is vascular in nature.

Radiologically the shape is round or oval with a smooth periphery (Fig. 20.3). If it is viewed from side is resembles a straight or slightly curved sausage. It may be homogenously radiopaque but more commonly has a appearance of laminations. A radiolucent center may be seen, which may represent the remaining patent portion of the vessels (Fig. 20.3).

Metastatic Calcification

In this calcium salts are precipitated in previous undamaged tissue. This precipitation is due to an excess of blood calcium and occurs particularly in such diseases as hyperthyroidism which depletes the bone of calcium and

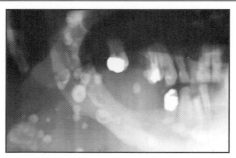

Fig. 20.3: Phleboliths was present.
(*Courtesy:* Dr Henrique Taglianetti)

causes a high level of blood calcium. The deposits of calcium occur in the kidney, lungs, gastric mucosa and blood vessels.

Ossification of the Stylohyoid Ligament

Ossification of stylohyoid is common and when it is associated with discomfort it is called as '*Eagle's syndrome*'. Ossification usually extends downward from the base of the skull and commonly occurs bilaterally. Bone tissue forms within segments of the stylohyoid ligament.

There is hard pointed structure over the tonsil. Vague pain on swallowing, turning the head and opening the mouth. Patient may describe earache, headache, dizziness or transient syncope which is caused by elongated styloid process impinging on glossopharyngeal nerve. Clinical finding without the history of neck trauma constitutes '*stylohyoid syndrome*'.

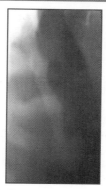

Fig. 20.4: Elongated styloid process with nodular mineralization pattern

Radiologically styloid process appears as long, lapping, thin, radiopaque process between ramus of mandible and mastoid process. Ossification of ligament roughly parallels the posterior border of the ramus. It appears as long, tapering, thin radiopaque process that is thicker at base and projects downward and forward (Fig. 20.4). As the ossification increases in length and girth, the outer cortex of it become evident as radiopaque band at the periphery.

Osteoma Cutis

These are sites of normal bone formation in abnormal locations. The lesion occur secondary to acne of long duration, developing in a scar or chronic inflammatory dermatosis.

Face is the most common site and tongue is the most common intraoral site. Size ranges from 0.1 to 5 cm and may be seen as single or multiple. Color may be normal or yellowish white. Needle when inserted is met with stone like resistance.

Radiologically smoothly outlined radiopaque washer-shaped image. They are very small, although size can range from 0.1 to 5 cm. It may be homogenous radiopaque or may have a radiolucent center that represent normal fatty marrow (Fig. 20.5).

Osteomas are occasionally removed for cosmetic reasons.

Myositis Ossificans

It is a condition in which fibrous tissue and heterotopic bone form within the interstitial tissue or muscle, as well as in associated tendons and ligaments. Secondary destruction and atrophy of the muscle occurs, as this fibrous tissue and bone interdigitate and separate the muscle fibers.

It can be localized myositis ossificans or traumatic myositis ossificans or progressive myositis ossificans or generalized myositis ossificans.

Localized Myositis Ossificans

It is also called as 'post-traumatic myositis ossificans' or 'solitary myositis'.

It is caused by acute or chronic trauma or heavy muscular strains caused by certain occupation or sports.

Site of trauma remains swollen, tender and painful much longer than expected. In some cases there is a mild discomfort

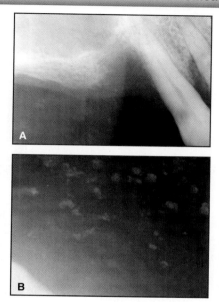

Figs 20.5A and B: Multiple miliary osteoma cutis. Patient with history of large quantity of acne for a long period of time. Periapical radiographs (A) showing evidence of ossifications in the soft tissues of the cheek. In B, the radiograph is obtained by placing the films in the vestibule, with low kilovolt exposure (*Courtesy:* Dr Filipe Ivan Daniel)

associated with a progressive limitation of motion. The overlying skin may be red and inflamed. The lesion may appear fixed or it may be freely movable on palpation (Fig. 20.6).

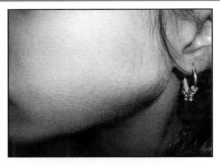

Fig. 20.6: Swelling seen in angle of mandible due to calcification

Orally it involves the muscles of face particularly masseter and temporal following single traumatic injury. Some difficulty in opening of the mouth.

Radiologically radiolucent band can be seen between the area of ossification and adjacent bone and heterotopic bone may lie along the long axis of the muscle. Faintly homogenous opacity. Delicate lacy or feathery internal structure of increased radiodensity develop indicating bone has formed. Sometimes it is accompanied by circumscribed cortical periphery. Margins are more radiopaque than the internal structure (Fig. 20.7). There is variation in shape from irregular oval to linear streaks running in the same direction as the normal muscle fibers.

Sufficient rest should be given with limitation of use. Excision after process becomes stationary.

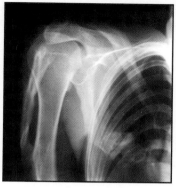

Fig. 20.7: Myosistis ossificans. See the increased radiodensity with margins more radiopaque than internal structure (*Courtesy:* Dr Bhaskar Patle, Lecturer Sharad Pawar Dental College, Wardha, India)

Progressive Myositis Ossificans

It is characterized by formation of bone in tendons and fascia with subsequent replacement of adjacent muscle by expanded bony mass. In some cases there is history of hereditary and familial pattern.

Soft tissue swelling that is tender and painful and may show redness and heat. Gradual increase in stiffness and limitation of motion of neck, chest and back and extremities. Ultimately entire groups of muscles become transformed into bone resulting in limitation of movements. The masseter muscle is frequently involved so that fixation of jaw occurs. The patient becomes transformed into a rigid organism called as 'petrified man'.

Radiologically there is evidence of dense osseous replacement of the greater part or whole of the muscle. Densities of heterotrophic bone vary widely. The bone that is laid down in the muscle does not show structure of normal bone but it is rather structureless mass of variable density. Lesion have smooth or irregular margins, lying in close relationship with the bone. The dense masses with passage of time tend to coalesce.

No effective treatment exists. Nodules that are traumatized and then ulcerate frequently should be excised.

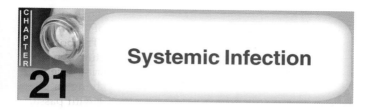

Systemic Infection

BACTERIAL INFECTION

Syphilis

It is also called as 'Lues'. It occurs most exclusively by venereal contact, in overcrowded living and primitive housing conditions.

It can be acquired (primary, secondary, tertiary and quaternary syphilis) or congenital.

Primary—lesion develop at the site of inoculation approximately 3 weeks after contact with infection. It is slightly raised, ulcerated, non-tender, non-bleeding, firm plaque which is usually rounded, indurated and with rolled raised edges. It is painless, unless super-infected. It disappears without therapy after 10 days. Regional lymph nodes become firm enlarged, rubbery in consistency and non-tender. Orally chancre has been described on lips (Fig. 21.1), in males (upper lip) and in females (lower lip), oral mucosa, lateral surface of tongue, soft palate, tonsillar area, pharyngeal lesion and gingiva.

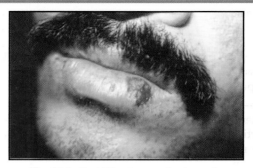

Fig. 21.1: Syphilitic ulcer on the lower lip

Secondary—organisms proliferate and spread by the way of blood stream to produce lesions else where. Usually appears within 3 to 6 weeks after primary lesion. When appear on skin, they manifest as fine macular or papular rash, sometimes accompanied by alopecia. Fever and generalized lymphadenopathy, which is painless, discrete and nonadherent to the surrounding tissues, may be seen. Mucus patches (small, smooth, erythematous areas or superficial grayish erosions found on mucous membrane of vulva, penis, or in oral cavity, on palate and tonsils. They are described as snail track ulcers), condyloma latum (grayish, moist, flat topped, extra large plaque which sometimes coalesce into larger plaques, found on moist mucocutaneous surfaces such as vulva, anus, scrotum, thigh and axilla), split papule (spilt papule is a double papule which occurs at skin folds and angle of mouth) is present. Orally mucus patches (appears as slightly raised grayish white lesions surrounded by erythematous base), snail track ulcers (confluence and coalescence of these glistening mucous patches gives rise to the so called 'snail track ulcers)' split papule (it is a raised papular lesion developed at the commissure of lip), condyloma latum (flat silver gray wart like papule, sometimes having ulcerated surface).

Tertiary—it may occur at any age from the third year upto the patient's life. Gumma is present which can be, i.e. central and cortical. Orally gumma can occur anywhere in the jaw but are more frequently on palate, mandible and tongue. Gumma may manifest as solitary, deep, punched out mucosal ulcer.

Leprosy (Hansen Disease)

It is a chronic infectious disease which has predilection for the skin, nerves and mucous membrane. It probably originated in tropic and spread to the east. Leprosy has always been considered in superstitious dread and the person suffering from leprosy was considered unclean and socially outcasted.

It is caused by the leprae bacillus, mycobacterium leprae, first observed by Hansen in 1868.

It can be tuberculoid, lepromatous, borderline tuberculoid, borderline lepromatous, polyneuritic, maculoanesthetic, indeterminate and erythema nodosum leprosum.

Incubation period of 2 to 5 years during which patient passes through silent or latent period.

Tuberculoid—lesions are hypopigmented, erythematous and flat or raised cutaneous lesions. Loss of eyebrows and eyelashes is prominent feature of later involvement.

Lepromatous leprosy—it is malignant form of the disease produced widespread involvement of body skin, peripheral nerves, mucous membrane, lymph nodes, eyes, skeleton tastes and other internal organs. It develops early as erythematous macules or papules (Fig. 21.3) without subsequently lead to progressive thickening of skin and the characteristic nodules. The borders of the lesion are ill defined and centers of the lesion are indurated and convex. Loss of lateral portion of eye brow is common. Much later, the skin of face and forehead become thickened and corrugated (leonine facies) and earlobe becomes pedunculous; nasal stiffness, epistaxis, hoarseness and saddle nose also occur. There is also presence of claw hand (Fig. 21.2) and leproma (Fig. 21.4).

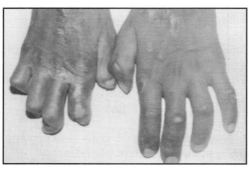

Fig. 21.2: Claw hand seen in leprosy patients

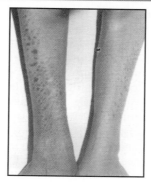

Fig. 21.3: Macular lesion seen on leg in patient of leprosy

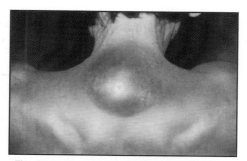

Fig. 21.4: Lepromas presented as well defined swelling at the neck of the patient

Erythema nodosum leprosum—they occur in lepromatous and borderline lepromatous patients, most frequently in the latter half of the initial year of treatment. Tender, inflamed subcutaneous nodules develop, usually in crops.

Orally depending on the type and duration of the disease, all patients with lepromatous leprosy show facial and oral manifestations and it is rare in tuberculoid and borderline leprosy. The lesions are macular or raised, well defined, hypopigmented, unhydrotic and hyperesthetic or anesthetic. Facial paralysis occurs while paralysis of the orbicularis muscle results in facial disfigurement, difficulties in phonation and mastication as well as drooling. Involvement of trigeminal nerve results in hypoesthesia and anesthesia. Collapse of the nose (saddle nose) is also observed (Fig. 21.5). Small tumor like masses called as lepromas develop on the tongue, lips or hard palate. These nodules have a tendency to breakdown and ulcerate. Gingival hyperplasia with loosening of teeth has been also reported.

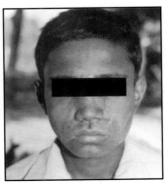

Fig. 21.5: Saddle nose and hypopigmentated lesion in leprosy

They get resolved either spontaneously or after treatment. Dapsone is effective choice of drug. Patient develops resistance to this drug then newer drugs such as clofazimine, rifampicine and prothionamide are used in combination to treat the disease.

Tuberculosis

It is a systemic infectious disease of worldwide prevalence and of varying clinical manifestations. It is an infectious granulomatous disease caused by acid-fast bacilli *Mycobacterium tuberculosis* or rarely, *Mycobacterium bovis*.

It can be miliary tuberculosis (wide involvement of many organs like kidney, liver and is called as miliary tuberculosis), Pott's disease (tubercular involvement of spine occurs in children) and scrofula (spreads by lymphatics to lymph nodes).

Patient may suffer episodes of fever and chills, easy fatigability and malaise. There may be gradual loss of weight accompanied by persistent cough with or without hemoptysis. Local symptoms depend upon the tissue or organs involved. Tubercular lymphadenitis (Fig. 21.6) may progress to acute abscess or remain as granulomatous lesion. In any case, swelling of neck is present which is tender, painful and often show inflammation of the overlying skin.

Ulcers are non-specific in their clinical presentation and for this reason they are overlooked by the clinician. The typical tuberculosis lesion is an irregular lesion with ragged undermined edges, minimum induration and often with yellowish granular base. The mucosa surrounding the ulcer

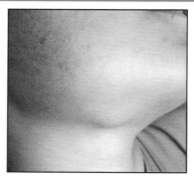

Fig. 21.6: Tubercular lymphadenitis seen as swelling in submandibular region

is inflamed and edematous. Tiny, single and multiple nodules called 'sentinel tubercle' may also be seen surrounding the ulcer.

Short-term chemotherapy, isoniazid (5 mg/kg with maximum of 300 mg daily or 15 mg/kg two to three times weekly) and rifampicin (10 gm/kg), ethambutol (25 gm/kg daily for no more than 2 months).

Actinomycosis

It is a chronic granulomatous suppurative and fibrous type of disease caused by anaerobic, gram positive, non-acid-fast bacteria. Most common are *Actinomycosis israeli, A. nasalundi, A. viscosus* and *A. odontolyticus.*

It can be cervicofacial, abdominal, pulmonary and cutaneous.

Cervicofacial form - the classical signs are chronic, low, grade persistence infection. The first sign of infection is characterized by the presence of a palpable mass. Mass is painless and indurated. Development of fistula is common. Skin surrounding the fistula is purplish. Several hard circumscribed tumor like swelling may develop and undergo breakdown, discharging a yellow fluid containing the characteristic submicroscopic sulfur granules.

Orally it produces swelling and induration of tissue. It may develop into one or more abscesses, which tend to discharge upon the skin surface liberating pus, which contains typical sulfur granules. Skin overlying abscess is purple red and indurate or fluctuant. It is common for sinus, through which the abscess has drained, to heal but due to chronicity, new abscesses are formed and perforate through skin surface. Infection may involve maxilla and mandible.

Radiologically, the radiographic appearance may resemble with apical rarefying osteitis. It may appear as an area of bone destruction, which resembles a dental cyst, with a well defined area of radiolucency with cortical lining of dense bone. Lamina dura is deficient at the apex of tooth. Scattered area of bone destruction, separated from one another by normal or sclerosed bone, is another manifestation.

Two-fold therapy including antibiotics and surgery is necessary. The lesion should be surgically removed and the surrounding area should be thoroughly debride.

Oral Myiasis

It is referred to the invasion of living tissues by the larvae of certain species of flies.

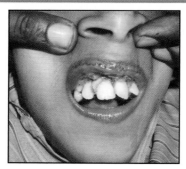

Fig. 21.7: Larvae are seen in upper anterior region in oral myiasis

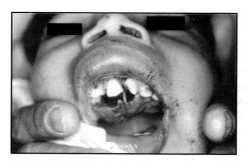

Fig. 21.8: Detachment of palate seen in mentally retarded patient due to larvae

It presents as an erythematous, edematous or granulomatous lesion. Itching or pain may be present. These lesions pulsate with movement of larvae. An opening is present from which larvae can come to surface of the lesion (Figs 21.7 and 21.8).

Surgical removal of larvae and irrigation of the tissue with hydrogen perioxide. Intestinal myiasis may require purgation with sodium sulphate or anti-helminthics.

Primary Herpes Simplex Infection

It is also called as 'Acute herpetic gingivostomatitis', 'Herpes labialis', 'Fever blister', 'Cold sore' and 'Infectious stomatitis'. It occurs in patients with no prior infection with HSV-I. HSV reaches nerve ganglion supplying the affected area, presumably along nerve pathways and remains latent until reactivated.

Prodromal symptoms precede local lesion by 1 to 2 days and it includes fever, headache, malaise, nausea, vomiting and within a few days, mouth becomes painful. There is also irritability, pain upon swallowing and regional lymphadenopathy. After this, small vesicles (Fig. 21.10), which are thin walled, surrounded by inflammatory base are formed. They quickly rupture leaving small, shallow, oval shaped discrete ulcers (Fig. 21.9). The base of the ulcer is covered with grayish white or yellow plaque. The margins of the sloughed lesions are uneven and are accentuated by bright red rimmed, well demarcated, inflammatory halos. The individual ulcer differs in size from 2-6 mm. As the disease progresses several lesions may coalesce, forming larger, irregular lesions, acute marginal gingivitis.

Topical anesthetics like lignocaine, dyclonine hydrochloride 0.5 percent, benzocaine hydrochloride are used. Topical anti-infective agents to prevent secondary infection are 0.2 percent chlorohexidine gluconate,

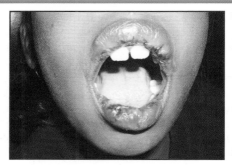

Fig. 21.9: Herpes simplex infection seen on
lip showing shallow ulcer

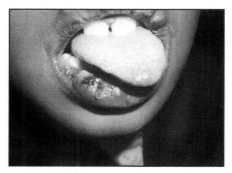

Fig. 21.10: Vesicle seen on tongue in herpes simplex infection

tetracycline mouth wash and elixir or diphenhydramine.
Acyclovir can be given.

Recurrent or Secondary Herpetic Infection

Recurrent infection is limited to localized portions of skin and mucous membrane.

It can be recurrent herpes labialis (RHL) or recurrent intraoral herpes (RIH) simplex infection. It is precipitated by surgery involving trigeminal ganglion as it remains latent in trigeminal ganglion. It is preceded by trauma to lips, fever, emotional upset and upper respiratory tract infection, sunburns, fatigue, menstruation and pregnancy, allergy and dental extraction.

If it occurs on lip, it is called as recurrent herpes labialis. If occurs intraorally it is called as recurrent intraoral herpes infection. In either location, lesion is preceded by tingling and burning sensation and feeling of tautness, swelling or slight soreness subsequent development of vesicle. It is accompanied by edema at the site of the lesion, followed by formation of clusters of small vesicles (Fig. 21.11). It range

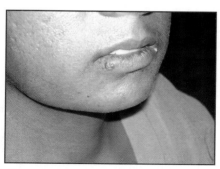

Fig. 21.11: Recurrent herpes labialis showing ulceration on the lip

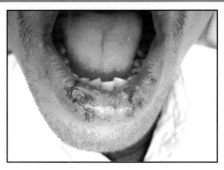

Fig. 21.12: Lip showing ulceration in RHL

from 1 to 3 mm in diameter, to 1 to 2 cm. But sometimes, it is large enough to cause disfigurement. These gray or white vesicles rupture quickly leaving small red ulcerations (Fig. 21.12), sometimes with slightly erythematous halo on lip covered by brownish crust on lips. The lesions gradually heal within 7-10 days and leave no scars.

Oral Acyclovir. Topical use of carbon oxolone useful in herpetic gingivostomatitis.

Measles

It is also called as 'Rubeola' or 'Morbilli'. It is an acute contagious dermatotropic viral infection, primarily affecting children and occurs many times in epidemic form.

Onset of fever, malaise, cough, conjunctivitis, photophobia, lacrimation and eruptive lesions of skin and oral mucosa. Otitis media and sore throat can occur. Skin eruption begins on face, in the hair line and behind the ear and spread to neck, chest, back and extremities. It appears as tiny red macules or papules which enlarge and coalesce to form blotchy discolored irregular lesions, which blanch on pressure. Fade away in 4 to 5 days with fine desquamation.

Oral lesions precede 2 to 3 days before cutaneous rash and are pathognomonic of this disease. Intraoral lesions are called as Koplik's spots which is small, irregularly shaped flecks which appear as bluish white specks surrounded by bright red margins. Generalized inflammation, congestion, swelling and focal ulceration of gingiva, palate, throat may occur (Fig. 21.13).

The patient should be isolated, if possible. Antiviral drug and vitamin A should be given.

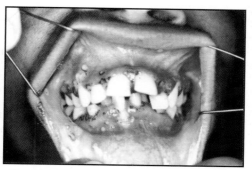

Fig. 21.13: Generalized inflammation of gingiva with some ulceration seen in measles

Varicella Zoster Infection

It is an acute disease caused by varicella zoster virus. After primary disease is healed, VZV becomes latent in the dorsal root ganglion of spinal nerve or extra-medullary ganglion of cranial nerve. VZV becomes reactivated causing lesions of localized herpes zoster.

It can be chickenpox (Varicella) and Shingles (herpes zoster) or zona.

Chickenpox

It is also called as 'Varicella'. It is an acute viral disease occurring in children and most commonly in winter and spring months.

It is characterized by prodromal occurrence of headache, nasopharyngitis and anorexia, followed by maculopapular or vesicular eruptions on skin and low grade fever. They occur in successive crops. The skin eventually ruptures, forming a superficial crust and heals by desquamation.

Orally small blister like lesions occasionally involve the oral mucosa chiefly buccal mucosa, tongue, gingiva, palate as well as the mucosa of pharynx. The mucosal lesion, initially a slightly raised vesicle with a surrounding erythema, ruptures soon after formation and forms a small eroded ulcer with red margins, closely resembling aphthous lesion.

Herpes Zoster

It is also called as 'Shingles' or 'Zona'. It is an acute infectious viral disease of extremely painful and incapacitating nature, characterized by inflammation of dorsal root ganglion, associated with vesicular eruptions of skin and mucous membrane of the area supplied by the affected sensory nerve.

Prodromal period of 2 to 4 days in which shooting pain, paresthesia, burning and tenderness appears along the course of affected nerve. Unilateral vesicles (Fig. 21.16) on an erythematous base appear in clusters, chiefly along the course of nerve and giving picture of a single dermatome involvement (Figs 21.14 and 21.15). Vesicle turns into scab in 1 week and healing takes place in 2 to 3 weeks. Nerves commonly affected are C3, T5, L1, L2 and 1st division of trigeminal nerve. It may affect motor nerve.

If Hutchison's sign (cutaneous zoster of the side of tip of nose) is present, then the probability of ocular involvement is more.

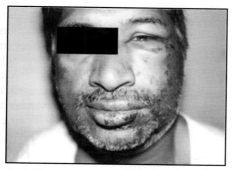

Fig. 21.14: Herpes zoster affecting trigeminal never on left side showing ulceration in the distribution of nerve

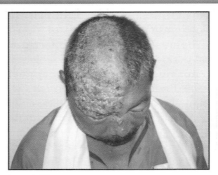

Fig. 21.15: Herpes zoster affecting the cranial nerve showing scab on the scalp

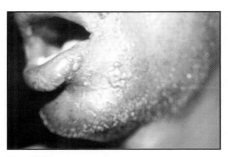

Fig. 21.16: Intact vesicle seen in herpes zoster

Orally it results from involvement of 2nd and 3rd divisions of trigeminal nerve. Lesions of oral mucosa are extremely painful. The lesions rupture to leave areas of erosion (Fig. 21.17).

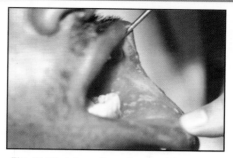

Fig. 21.17: Intraorally rupture vesicle seen in
case of herpes zoster patient

It is managed by acyclovir 800 mg five times daily which is associated with significantly accelerated healing within 48 hours of the onset of rash. Topical capsaicin 0.025 percent four times a day has been suggested for temporary relief of neuralgia following herpes zoster infection (Fig. 21.18).

Coxsackievirus Infection

They are RNA retroviruses and are named after town in upper New York where they were first discovered. They are divided into 2 groups.
- Type A - 24 types
- Type B - 6 types

Herpangina

It is also called as 'Apthous pharyngitis', 'vesicular pharyngitis'. A4 causes majority of the cases. A4 to A10 and

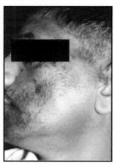

Fig. 21.18: Herpes zoster after treatment showing healed vesicle

A16 to A22 have also been implicated. It appears to be transmitted from one person to another through contact.

Initially, generalized symptoms of fever, chills, headache, anorexia, prostration, abdominal pain and sometimes vomiting. Sore throat, dysphagia and occasionally, sore mouth can occur. Lesion starts as punctuate macule which evolves into papules and vesicles. Within 24 to 48 hours, vesicles get ruptured forming small 1 to 2 mm ulcers. Ulcers show a grey base and inflamed periphery (Fig. 21.19).

Self limiting and supportive treatment by proper hydration and topical anesthetic, when eating or swallowing is difficult.

Acute Lymphonodular Pharyngitis

It is caused by A10 and is same as herpangina. Yellow-white nodules appear that do not progress to vesicles or ulcers. It is self limiting and only supportive care is indicated.

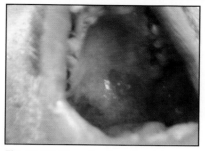

Fig. 21.19: Ulceration in soft palate occur due to Coxsackies virus infection

Hand Foot Mouth Disease

It is caused by A16, A5, A7, A9, A10, B2 and B5. It is characterized by appearance of maculopapular, exanthematous and vesicular lesions of skin, particularly involving the hands, feet, legs, arms and occasionally buttocks.

Orally a sore mouth with refusal to eat is one of the most common findings in this disease. The tongue may become red and edematous.

No specific treatment is necessary since the disease is self limiting and generally regresses within one to two weeks.

FUNGAL INFECTION

Histoplasmosis

It is also called as 'Darling's disease'. It is caused by *Histoplasma capsulatum*.

It can be acute primary histoplasmosis, progressive disseminated histoplasmosis.

Acute primary histoplasmosis - chronic low grade fever, malaise, headache and productive cough. Primary infection is mild, manifesting as self limited pulmonary disease that heals to leave fibrosis and calcification.

Progressive disseminated histoplasmosis - it is manifested by hepatosplenomegaly and lymphadenopathy.

Oral lesions are common in the progressive disseminated form. Patient may complain of sore throat, painful chewing, hoarseness, difficulty in swallowing. Oral lesions are nodular, ulcerative or vegetative. Ulcerated area covered by non-specific gray membrane and is indurated.

It is managed by ketoconazole - 6 to 12 months. Severe form - Amphotericin B, IV.

Mucormycosis

It is also called as 'Phycomycosis'.

It is caused by saprophyte fungus. More common in patients with decreased resistance, due to diseases like diabetes, tuberculosis, renal failure, leukemia, cirrhosis and in severe burn cases.

It can be superficial, or visceral. Rhinomaxillary form begins with inhalation of fungus by susceptible individual. Infection usually arise in lateral wall of nose and maxillary sinus; may rapidly spread by arterial invasion to involve the orbit, palate, maxillary alveolus and ultimately the cavernous sinus and brain through hematogenous spread and may cause death. There is increased lethargy,

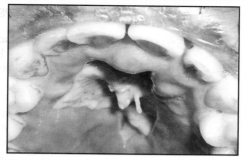

Fig. 21.20: Mucormycosis showing ulceration in the palate

progressive neurologic deficit and ultimately death. There is appearance of a reddish black nasal turbinate and septum. Nasal discharge caused by necrosis of nasal turbinate.

Ulceration of palate, due to necrosis and invasion of palatal vessels (Fig. 21.20). Ulcer may be seen on gingivae, lip and alveolar bone. It is large and deep, causing denudation of underlying bone.

Radiologically paranasal sinus may reveal mucoperiosteal thickening of the involved sinus. With disease progression, there is increased nodularity and soft tissue thickening, usually mimics a tumor on radiographical examination. Surgical debridment is the treatment of choice. Systemic Amphotericin. Control of predisposing factors such as diabetes.

Systemic Disease Manifested in Jaw

AIDS

It is a devastating fatal disease which is in epidemic form throughout the world. It is an incurable viral STD which is cause by human immune deficiency virus. It stands for:

- A -Acquired, i.e. contagious not inherited.
- I - Immune, i.e. power to receive disease.
- D - Deficiency.
- S - Syndrome, i.e. number of signs and complains indicative of particular disease.

  It is caused by HIV (human immunodeficiency virus).

DEFINITION

WHO has given following definition of AIDS.

One or more opportunistic infections listed in clinical features that are at least moderately indicative of underlying cellular immune deficiency.

- Absence of all known underlying causes of cellular immune deficiency (other than HIV infection) and absence of all other causes of reduced resistance reported to be associated with at least one of those opportunistic diseases.

AIDS Related Complex

For clinical and research studies, persons exhibiting complex clinical problems and immunological or hematological abnormalities on the laboratory tests, have been classified as having AIDS related complex. ARC requires any two or more symptoms and two or more abnormal laboratory findings. It must be present for at least 3 months.

Symptoms present are lymphadenopathy, weight loss of 15 lbs or 10 percent of body weight, fever of 38.5°C which is intermittent or continuous, diarrhea, fatigue and malaise and night sweats. Lab finding includes decreased number of T helper cell, decreased ratio of T helper cells to T suppressor cells, anemia or leukopenia or thrombocytopenia or lymphopenia, increased serum globulin level, and decreased blastogenic response of lymphocytes to mitogen, increased level of circulating immune complex. cutaneous anergy to multiple the skin test antigens. Anergy is impaired or inability to react to skin antigens.

Clinical Features

Protozoan and helminthes infection - Cryptosporidiosis (intestinal) causing diarrhea for over one month. The most common opportunistic infection is by pneu-mocystis carinii which causes pneumonia.

Fungal infection: Candidiasis causing esophagitis. Cryptococcosis causing CNS infection.

Bacterial infections: *Mycobacterium avian* intra-cellulare causing infection disseminated beyond lung and lymph node. *Mycobacterium tuberculosis* causing tuberculosis.

Viral infections: Cytomegalovirus, causing infection in the internal organs other than liver, spleen and lymph nodes. Herpes simplex virus, causing chronic mucocutaneous infection with ulcers persisting more than one month.

Malignancy: Kaposi's sarcoma and squamous cell carcinoma. Lymphoma limited to bronchi and non-Hodgkin's lymphoma.

Oral Manifestations

Oral manifestations of HIV disease are common and include oral lesions and novel presentations of previously known opportunistic diseases (Fig. 22.1). The presence of these

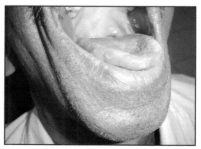

Fig. 22.1: Ulceration similar aphthous ulcer seen on the tongue in HIV patient

lesions may be an early diagnostic indicator of immunodeficiency and HIV infection, may change the classification
of the stage of HIV infection and is a predictor of the
progression of HIV disease. 95 percent of AIDS patients
have head and neck lesion and about 55 percent have
important oral manifestation.

The most common presentations include pseudomembranous and erythematous candidiasis, which are
equally predictive of the development of AIDS and angular
cheilitis (Fig. 22.2).

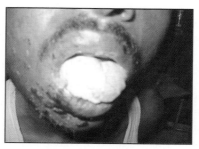

Fig. 22.2: Pseudomembranous type of
candidiasis seen in HIV patient

Recurrent herpes labialis: It mainly appear as herpes labialis
and recurrent intraoral herpes. Herpes labialis occurs as
characteristic lip lesion consisting of vesicles on an
erythematous base that heals within 7 to 10 days.

Herpes zoster: The occurrence of unilateral vesicles that break
and scab is characteristic of this infection (Fig. 22.3).

Cytomegalovirus infection: It has got predilection for salivary glands because many HIV infected patients have xerostomia.

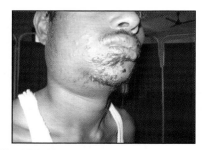

Fig. 22.3: Herpes zoster lesion in HIV patient

Salivary gland disease: It can present as xerostomia with or without salivary gland enlargement. Reports describe salivary gland enlargement in children and adults with HIV infection usually involving the parotid gland.

Hairy leukoplakia: Oral hairy leukoplakia, which presents as a non-movable, corrugated or "hairy" white lesion on the lateral margins of the tongue occurs in all risk groups for HIV infections, although less commonly in children than in adults (Fig. 22.4). Epstein Barr virus has identified in these lesions. It occur unilaterally or bilaterally on the lateral border of tongue. It can also occur on dorsum of the tongue, buccal mucosa, and floor of mouth, retromolar area and soft palate. There is characteristic corrugated and white appearance (Fig. 22.4). It does not rub off and may resemble the keratotic lesion.

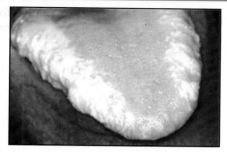

Fig. 22.4: Hairy leukoplakia showing corrugated and white appearance on the tongue

Kaposi's sarcoma: It is also called as 'angioreticulo-endothelioma'. It is the most common tumor associated with AIDS and occurs in 1/3rd of AIDS patients. It begins as multinucleated neoplastic process that manifests as multiple red or purple macules and in more advanced stage, a nodule occurring on the skin or mucosal surface. It can appear as a red, blue, or purplish lesion. It may be flat or raised solitary or multiple. The lesions may enlarge, ulcerate and become infected.

Atypical periodontal disease: periodontal disease is a fairly common problem in both asymptomatic and symptomatic HIV-infected patients. It can take two forms: the rapid and severe condition called necrotizing ulcerative periodontitis and it's associated and possibly precursor condition called linear gingival erythema. It often occur in clean mouths where there is very little plaque or calculus to account for the gingivitis. The ulcers heal, leaving the gingival papillae with a characteristic cratered appearance. Necrotizing ulcerative periodontitis may present as rapid loss of supporting bone and soft tissue. Teeth may loosen and eventually fall out, but uninvolved sites can appear healthy.

Management

Various treatment modalities used are interferon, thymic replacement therapy, lymphokines and cytokines, bone marrow transplantation, monoclonal antibodies therapy, pharmacological immunomodulation, intravenous immunoglobulin therapy, antiviral drug (HPA-23, aidothymidine, cyclosporin).

DISEASES OF RED BLOOD CELLS

Sickle Cell Anemia

It is autosomal dominant. It was first described by Herrick in 1910. This is the most common type of hemoglobinopathy in which there is a substitution of amino acid glutamine on position 6 present in the chain of the HbA, by valine; giving rise to an abnormal Hb, i.e. hemoglobin S. In homozygous individuals, whole of HbA is replaced by HbS and this is known as 'sickle cell disease' and in heterozygous individuals, only 50 percent of HbA is replaced by HbS and this is known as 'sickle cell trait'.

There is fatigue, weakness and shortness of breath. Severe abdominal pain, muscle and joint pain, at high temperature which may result in circulatory collapse. There is increased susceptibility to infection. Most of persons expire before the age of 40 years. Sickle cell crisis - there is a long quit spell of hemolytic latency occasionally punctated by exacerbations called as sickle cell crisis.

The oral mucosa will show pallor and jaundice. There may be delayed eruption and hypoplasia of the dentition, secondary to their general development. This may be due to hypovascularity of the bone marrow secondary to thrombosis.

Radiologically because of chronic increased erythropoietic activity and marrow hyperplasia, there is loss of trabeculation of the jaw bone resulting in a mild to severe generalized osteoporosis and appearance of large irregular marrow spaces. The trabeculae in between the roots of teeth may appear as horizontal rows creating 'step ladder' like effect. Skull radiographs show an unusual appearance, with perpendicular trabeculation radiating outward from the inner table producing a 'hair on end' pattern.

It is managed by folic acid - regular folic acid supplement (5 mg/daily) is given to support the greatly increased erythropoietin. Blood transfusion should be given during crisis only. Routinely it should be avoided, because it increases the viscosity of blood.

Thalassemia

It is also called as 'Cooley's anemia', 'Mediterranean anemia' and 'erythroblastic anemia'. Either alpha or beta globulin genes may be affected. It is autosomal dominant.

It can be α thalassemia (absence of a alpha chain), beta thalassemia (absence of beta chains), thalassemia major or homozygous β-thalassemia, thalassemia intermedia, thalassemia minor or thalassemia trait (when the patient heterozygous).

The patient first presents with pallor of skin, fever, chills, malaise, generalized weakness, prominent cheek bone and mild hepatosplenomegaly. Bone marrow hyperplasia in early life may produce frontal head bossing and there may be marked overdevelopment of malar bone which is associated with a shot nose having a depressed bridge giving the appearance of mongoloid.

Orally there is excessive overgrowth of maxilla causing excessive lacrimation and nasal stuffness. The oral mucosa is pale and has a lemon yellow tint because of chronic jaundice. Due to high concentration of iron, discoloration of dentin and enamel maybe evident. There is also saddle nose, prominent malar bone and pneumatization of maxillary sinus. As a result of these skeletal changes, the upper lip is retracted giving the child a 'chip munk' facies.

Radiologically the lamina dura is thin and the roots of the teeth may be short. There is thinning of the crypt of developing teeth. The marrow spaces are large and the trabeculae are large and course. Skull is thickened as a result of increased width of the dipole space between the outer and inner tables of the vault. This occurs due to proliferation of the hemopoietic tissue. The trabeculae joining the inner and outer table of the skull are readily arranged calcified spicules which appear as calcified hair extending between the inner and outer tables, which is called as 'hair on end' appearance (Fig. 22.5).

Blood transfusion, splenectomy, chelating agent, folic acid.

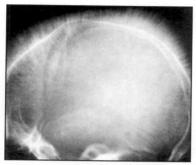

Fig. 22.5: Typical hair on end appearance seen in thalassemia patient
(*Courtesy:* Dr AK Ganju, Clinical Hematologist, Nagpur, India)

Iron Deficiency Anemia

Iron is essential for synthesis of 'hem' portion of hemoglobin. Iron deficiency anemia is caused by imbalance between iron intake and loss or inadequate utilization.

The patient experiences tiredness, headache, paresthesia and lack of concentration. Nails become brittle, flattened and often show spoon shape (koilonychia). There may be tingling and pins and needle sensation in the extremities. Some patients develop pharyngeal mucosal thickening and mucosal web formation, giving rise to dysphagia.

In iron deficiency there is pallor of oral mucosa and gingiva. The generalized atrophy of oral mucosa both in tongue and buccal mucosa occurs. There is redness, soreness or burning of tongue. There is softening of epithelium which leads to linear ulceration of the skin, extending up to and beyond the muco-cutaneous junction. In some cases there may be gingival enlargement (Fig. 22.6).

It is managed by giving iron supplement.

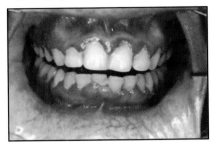

Fig. 22.6: Gingival enlargement seen in iron deficiency anemia. As such this is rare finding

Megaloblastic Anemia

This results due to deficiency of vitamin B_{12} and folate or both, resulting in disordered cell proliferation leading to megaloblastic anemia.

It is caused by folate deficiency or vitamin B_{12} deficiency.

There are symptoms of anemia like weakness, loss of appetite and palpitations. In severe cases, skin may show faint lemon yellow tint and spleen may be palpable. Many cases show paresthesia of finger and toes and dementia may also be seen.

Orally burning sensation in tongue, hypersensitivity, paresthesia and later dryness of the mouth. Atrophy of filiform and fungiform papillae leads to (Fig. 22.7) completely atrophic smooth fiery red surface of tongue (Hunter's glossitis). Angular cheilitis and dysphagia due to pharyngitis and esophagitis.

Blood transfusion, vitamin B$_{12}$, folic acid should be given.

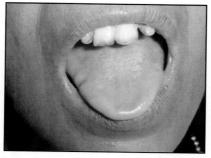

Fig. 22.7: Atrophy of filiform papillae occur in megaloblastic anemia

DISEASE OF WHITE BLOOD CELLS

Cyclic Neutropenia

It is also called as 'periodic neutropenia'. It is a rare disorder characterized by periodic or cyclic diminution in circulating neutrophils due to failure of stem cells of bone marrow. It is also called as periodic neutropenia. The patient is healthy between neutropenic periods; but at regular intervals, the absolute neutrophils count falls below 500/mm^3.

The patients manifest fever, sore throat, stomatitis and regional lymphadenopathy as well as headache, arthritis, cutaneous infection and conjunctivitis.

Orally severe gingivitis and painful ragged ulcers (Fig. 22.8) that have a core like center are found on the lip, tongue, palate, gums and buccal mucosa which heal after about two weeks with scarring. Isolated painful ulcer may occur which correspond to the period of neutropenia.

There is no specific treatment and monitoring the patient for infection during neutropenic period and vigorous early management of infection.

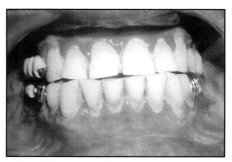

Fig. 22.8: Severe gingivitis seen in cases of cyclic neutropenia showing ulceration

Lazy Leukocyte Syndrome

It is a result of loss of chemotactic function of the neutrophils. The neutrophils present in the blood can not migrate to the site of tissue injury although phagocytic and bactericidal activities are normal.

The most common clinical manifestations are stomatitis, otitis media and bronchitis.

Orally gingivitis and stomatitis are common oral finding of this disorder. In some cases periodontal disease may be present.

Chediak-Higashi Syndrome

It is a congenital autosomal recessive defect of granulocytes and melanocytes. Abnormal granules are seen in all blood granulocytes resulting in decreased chemotactic and bactericidal activity, although phagocytosis remains intact.

The characteristic clinical feature of this disease consists of oculocutaneous albinism, photophobia, nystagmus and recurrent infections of the respiratory tract and sinuses.

Orally ulcerations of the oral mucosa, severe gingivitis and glossitis are the common oral lesions. There may be rarely loss of teeth due to periodontal disease.

PLATELET DISORDERS

Idiopathic Thrombocytopenic Purpura

It is also called as 'Werlhof's disease', 'purpura hemo-rrhagic' and 'primary thrombocytopenic purpura'. It is a disease in which there is an abnormal reduction in the number of circulating blood platelets with normal or raised number of megakaryocytes in the bone marrow.

Thrombocytopenic purpura is characterized by spontaneous appearance of purpuric hemorrhagic lesions of skin, which vary in size from tiny red pin point petechiae to large purplish ecchymoses and sometimes, even massive hematoma. Epistaxis, hematuria and melena are common findings.

Orally the first manifestation of the disease can be seen in oral cavity in the form of excessive bleeding after tooth extraction. It appears as numerous tiny, grouped clusters of reddish spots, only a millimeter or less in diameter (Figs 22.10 and 22.11). Petechiae do not blanch on pressure which is the distinguishing feature between purpura and telangiectasia. In severe cases, extensive spontaneous gingival bleeding may be seen and this may form foci of secondary infection (Fig. 22.9).

Corticosteroids, splenectomy, transfusion, local hemostatic.

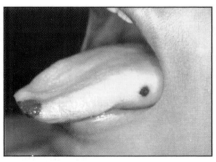

Fig. 22.9: Hemorrhagic lesion seen from the tongue in idiopathic thrombocytopenic purpura

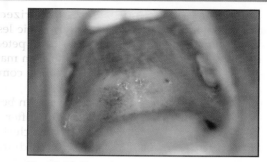

Fig. 22.10: Purpuric lesion seen on the soft palate

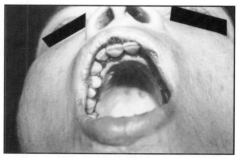

Fig. 22.11: Spontaneous bleeding seen from the gingiva
in idiopathic thrombocytopenic purpura

Secondary Thrombocytopenic Purpura

It is caused by drugs (barbiturates, analgesics (phenylbutazone and Salicylates), antihistamine (diphenhydramine
hydrochloride), myelosuppressive agents used in neoplastic

disease), infections (viral and bacterial), malignancy (carcinoma, leukemia, sarcoma, lymphoma, Hodgkin's disease), metabolic (uremia, megaloblastic anemia), bone marrow replacement, myelofibrosis, radiation therapy and systemic lupus erythematous.

They are similar to idiopathic thrombocytopenic purpura (Fig. 22.12). Here, prognosis is much better provided the underlying cause is removed and transfusion is given as required.

Eliminating the cause, remaining treatment is same as that of ITP.

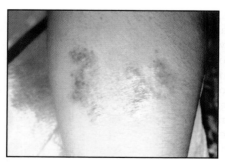

Fig. 22.12: Hemorrhagic lesion seen on hand of the patient seen in purpura

Disturbances in Lipid Metabolism

Lipids are a heterogeneous group of organic compounds which are relatively insoluble in water but, soluble in solvent such as ether, chloroform and benzene.

Hand - Schuller - Christian Disease

It is also called as *'multifocal eosinophilic granuloma'* *'chronic disseminated histiocytosis X'* or *'xanthomatosis*. It is characterized by widespread skeletal and extraskeletal lesions and chronic clinical course. It is result of error in the metabolism of cholesterol and its esters.

Classic triad of single or multiple areas of punched out bone destruction in skull, unilateral or bilateral Exophthalmos and diabetes insipidus. Involvement of facial bone which is commonly associated with soft tissue swelling and tenderness causing facial asymmetry.

Sore mouth with or without ulcerative lesion, halitosis, gingivitis and suppuration. An unpleasant taste, loose and sore teeth with precocious exfoliation and failure of healing of tooth socket following extraction. Loss of supporting alveolar bone mimics advanced periodontal disease.

Radiologically bone lesion usually seen in membrane bone but can occur in long bones and the mandible. The skull lesion may be small or large, single or multiple and they may occur anywhere but anterior portion of the vault and the floor of anterior and middle cranial fossa is commonest site. The lesions are entirely destructive, so there is radiolucency which usually sharply defined but with no cortical margin. It is well define at periphery with punch out appearance (Figs 22.13 and 22.14). Margins are smooth or somewhat irregular. Destruction of periodontal bone support of one or more teeth especially in the posterior areas while producing virtually no resorption of tooth roots. The result is often a distinctive radiographic appearance of 'teeth

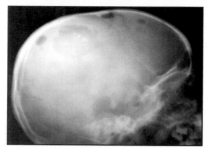

Fig. 22.13: Punched out lesion seen in histiocytosis X in the skull

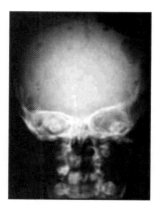

Fig. 22.14: Histiocytosis X. Note the punched radiolucent image seen in the skull (*Courtesy:* Dr Praveen Lambade, Associate Professor, CDC College, Rajnandgaon, India)

standing in space (floating teeth appearance) in the region superior to the mandibular canal.

Prognosis of this disease is good and half of the patients undergo spontaneous remission over a period of a year. It is usually treated by curettage or excision of lesion. The lesions which are inaccessible are treated by irradiation.

Eosinophilic Granuloma

This term was introduced by Lichtenstein and Jaffe in 1940. It is also called as 'unifocal eosinophilic granuloma'. It is the lesion of bone which is primarily histiocytes proliferation with an abundance of eosinophilic leukocytes by no intra- or extracellular lipid accumulation.

There may be local pain which may be dull and steady, swelling and tenderness. General malaise and fever may accompany the eosinophilic granuloma of bone. Lesion is destructive and well demarcated, roughly round or oval in shape.

Orally there is loss of superficial alveolar bone often mimicking juvenile periodontitis. Gingivitis and bleeding gingiva, pain or ulceration is present. Loosening and sloughing of teeth often occurs after destruction of alveolar bone.

Radiologically eosinophilic granuloma may be solitary or multiple and the lesions are circular or elliptical in shape. It is moderately well defined at its radiographic periphery. The lesion in the jaw has fairly discrete borders, which are rarely hyperostotic.

It is usually treated with curettage and X-ray therapy. Symptoms usually subside within 2 weeks after treatment.

Hyperpituitarism

It results from hyperfunction of anterior lobe of pituitary gland, most significantly with increased production of growth hormone.

It can be gigantism (if the increase occurs before the epiphysis of the long bone are closed) and acromegaly - if the increase occurs later in life after epiphysis closure.

Gigantism - generalized overgrowth of most tissue in childhood (Fig. 22.15). Most of the soft tissue and bones respond to the excess hormone by enlarging. Excessive generalized skeletal growth. Patient may often have of height to 7 to 8 feet. Patients achieve monstrous size because of tumors of the pituitary gland.

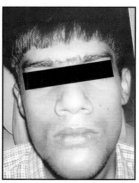

Fig. 22.15: Patient having acromegaly showing more growth at condylar center

Acromegaly - bone overgrowth and thickening of the soft tissue cause a characteristic coarsening of facial features termed acromegaly. Hand and feet become large, with clubbing of the toes and fingers due to enlargement of the tufts of the terminal phalanges. There is temporal headache, photophobia and reduction in vision. The terminal phalanges of the hands and feets become large and the ribs also increase in size.

Teeth in gigantism are proportional to the sized of jaw and the rest of the body and root may be longer than normal. The teeth become spaced, partly because of enlargement of the tongue and party because upper teeth are situated on the inner aspect of the lower dental arch, due to dispro-portionate enlargement of the two jaws. Mandibular condylar growth is very prominent. Overgrowth of mandible leading to prognathism. In some cases the growth at the condyle exceeds that of the alveolar processes, so that increased in vertical depth of the ramus is greater than that of the body of the jaw, consequently the upper and lower teeth fail to come into proper occlusion.

Radiologically enlargement of sella tursica, enlargement of paranasal sinus (Fig. 22.16) and excessive pneumatization of temporal bone squamous and petrous ridge. Diffuse thickening of outer table of skull. Enlargement and distortion of the pituitary fossa. Increased tooth size especially root due to secondary cemental hyperplasia. Diastema between teeth due to lengthening of dental arch. Increase in thickness and height of alveolar process.

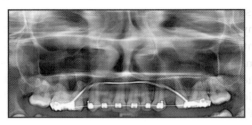

Fig. 22.16: Enlarged maxillary sinus in case of hyperpituitarism

Trans-sphenoidal surgery may result in cure of GH excess especially in patients with macroadenoma. Octreotide, a long acting analogue of somatostatin, lowers GH. It is administered as subcutaneous insulin 2 to 3 times/day. Dopamine antagonists are also used.

Hypopituitarism

It results due to reduced secretion of pituitary hormone which may occur due to pituitary adenoma that compresses the pituitary gland. It results in pituitary dwarfism. Pathologic changes can results from a variety of pituitary gland malfunction. Total absence of all pituitary secretions is known as panhypopituitarism. Hypopituitarism which commences after puberty is called as 'Simmond's disease'.

The underdevelopment is symmetrical, individual is very small and in some cases there may be a disproportional shortening of the long bones.

Marked failure of development of maxilla and mandible with lack of condylar growth with short ramus and this can lead to severe malocclusion and crowding of the teeth. In case of hypofunction this gland, tooth eruption is hampered. The dental arch is smaller than normal and thus can not accommodate all the teeth resulting in crowding and subsequent malocclusion.

Radiologically complete absence of third molar bud. Roots of teeth are short and apices are wide open and pulp canal toward the apex. There is loss of alveolar bone.

It is usually directed towards removal of the cause or replacement of the pituitary hormone or those of its target glands.

Hyperthyroidism

It is also called as 'thyrotoxicosis' and it is a syndrome in which there is excessive production of thyroxin in thyroid gland. It is associated with diffuse toxic goiter and less frequently with toxic nodular goiter or toxic adenoma.

It is caused by exophthalmic goiter, toxic adenoma, ectopic thyroid tissue, Graves disease, multinodular goiter, thyroid adenoma.

Thyroid is diffusely enlarged, smooth, possible asymmetrical and nodular (Fig. 22.17), a thrill may be present, may be tender. Abdomen, liver and spleen may be enlarged. There are also nervousness, fine tremors, and muscle weakness, mood swings from depression to extreme euphoria, emotional liability, hyper-reflexia, ill sustained clonus, proximal myopathy, bulbar myopathy and periodic paralysis.

Advanced rate of dental development and early eruption with premature loss of primary teeth. Generalized decrease in bone density or loss of some areas of edentulous alveolar bone. Early jaw development and alveolar bone atrophy.

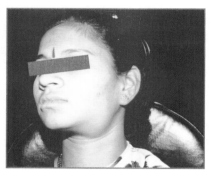

Fig. 22.17: Swelling of thyroid gland in the neck
(*Courtesy:* Dr Lambade, CDC, Rajnandgaon, India)

Radiologically in older children and adults well marked generalized osteoporosis is sometime appears but it is not reveal in the jaw. In some cases there may be alveolar resorption and in some cases there may be greater density of the trabeculae.

Antithyroid drugs should be given.

Hypothyroidism

It is caused by insufficient secretion of thyroxin by the thyroid gland.

It can be cretinism (if failure of hormone occurs in infancy), juvenile myxedema (if it occurs in childhood) and myxedema (after the puberty).

Cretinism and juvenile myxedema - hoarse cry, constipation, feeding problems in neonates. Retarded mental and physical growth occurs. Delayed fusion of all body epiphysis and delayed ossification of paranasal sinus, partially pneumatization. There is protuberant abdomen with umbilical hernia. The hairs are sparse and brittle, the finger nails are brittle and the sweat glands are atrophic.

Myxedema - it may include weakness, fatigue, cold intolerance, and lethargy, dryness of skin, headache, menorrhagia, and anorexia. In later stage there is slowing of intellectual and motor activity, absence of sweating, modest weight gain, constipation, peripheral edema, pallor, hoarseness, decreased sense of taste and smell, muscle cramps, aches and pains, dyspnea, anginal pain and deafness. Dull expressionless face, periorbital edema, sparse hair and skin that feels droughty to touch.

Orally in cretinism and juvenile myxedema dental development delayed and primary teeth slow to exfoliate. Enamel hypoplasia can also be seen. Maxilla is overdeveloped and mandible is underdeveloped. Retarded condylar growth leads to characteristic micrognathia and open bite relationship. Tongue is enlarged by edema fluid and due to it tongue may protruded continuously and such protrusion may lead to malocclusion of teeth.

Radiologically delayed closing of the fontanels and epiphysis, numerous wormian bones (accessory bone in the sutures). There is transverse line of increased density involving the metaphysical regions. There is thinning of lamina dura. Delayed dental eruption, short tooth root.

It is managed by thyroid preparation like levothyroxin.

Hyperparathyroidism

It is an endocrine disorder in which there is an excess of circulating parathyroid hormone. Excess PTH stimulates osteoclast to mobilize calcium from skeleton leading to hypercalcemia in addition to PTH increased renal tubular re-absorption of calcium.

It can be primary, secondary, tertiary ectopic.

Renal calculi are common and hematuria, back pain, urinary tract infection and hypertension are common. Peptic ulcer, psychiatric effect like emotional instability, bone and joint pain, and sometime pathologic fractures occurs. Gastrointestinal difficulties such as anorexia, nausea, vomiting and crampy pain may be present. Bone deformities occur such as bending of long bone occasional fracture and collapse of vertebrae and formation of pigeon chest.

Orally there is gradual loosening drifting and loss of teeth, malocclusion. There is pathological fracture of bone. Cystic lesion involving jaws are seen over 10 percent of cases.

Radiologically bone matrix contains less than normal amounts of calcium producing unusually radiolucent skeletal image. There is lack of normal contrast in the radiograph resulting in over all grayness, often associated with a granular appearance in the bone. The rarefaction is of homogeneous nature and there may be normal, granular or ground glass appearance.

Brown tumor (Fig. 22.18): It may develop peripherally or centrally. It appears radiographically as ill-defined radiolucency called as brown tumor, as gross specimen is brown or reddish brown. In it, trabeculae are completely missing. It may occur in pelvis, ribs or femur but are most commonly found in facial bones and jaws. These lesions may be multiple within the single bone or they may be polyostotic. They appear as unilocular or multilocular with

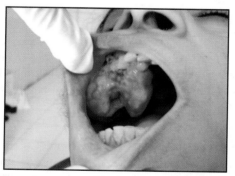

Fig. 22.18: Brown tumor, present in the oral cavity, drifting the associated teeth (*Courtesy:* Dr Amit Parate, Lecturer, Govt. Dental College and Hospital, Nagpur, India)

variably defined margin and may produce cortical expansion (Figs 22.19 and 22.20).

If the alveolus is severely affected the teeth may become mobile and migrate (Fig. 22.20). The radiopaque cortical plate outlining the bones and anatomic regions may be thinned or lost entirely. Loss of lamina dura which may be

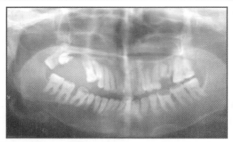

Fig. 22.19: Brown tumor, presented as irregular bone loss in upper posterior region. Note the drifting of the associated teeth (*Courtesy:* Dr Amit Parate, Lecturer, Govt. Dental College and Hospital, Nagpur, India)

seen around one tooth or all remaining teeth. It may be complete or partial.

It often regresses without surgery and the rarefaction disappears. Surgical excision of adenoma.

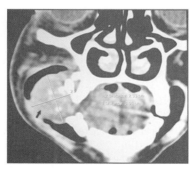

Fig. 22.20: CT image of brown tumor (arrow) (*Courtesy:* Dr Amit Parate, Lecturer, Govt. Dental College and Hospital, Nagpur, India)

Hypoparathyroidism

It is an uncommon condition in which there is insufficient secretion of parathyroid hormone.

It can lead to tetany in the form of carpopedal spasm of the wrist and ankle joint. Stiffness in hands, feet and lips. There is also paresthesia of hand feet and around the mouth. Tingling in the circumoral area, fingers ad toes.

There is hypoplasia of enamel, delayed eruption, external root resorption and root dilacerations. There is also blunting of molar roots. Chvostek sign (a sharp tap over the facial nerve in front of ear causes muscle twitching of facial muscle around the mouth) is positive. Chronic candidiasis is also some time present.

Radiologically there is calcification of basal ganglion which appears flocculent and paired with the cerebral hemisphere on PA view. Radiograph of jaw may reveal enamel hypoplasia, external root resorption, delayed eruption or root calcification.

Supplemental calcium and vitamin D depending on severity of the hypocalcemia and the nature of the associated signs and symptoms.

GRANULOMATOUS DISORDERS
Wegner's Granulomatosis

It is a disease of unknown etiology which basically involves the vascular, renal and respiratory systems. It is a granulomatous involvement of blood vessels resulting in necrosis of tissue.

The most common symptom of Wegner's granulomatosis is nasal stuffiness with chronic discharge, which is sometimes bloody. Patient soon develops cough, hemoptysis, fever and joint pains. There is also presence of rhinitis, sinusitis and otitis or ocular symptoms. There are also non-specific symptoms of malaise, arthralgia and weight loss. Hemorrhagic or vesicular skin lesions are also commonly present. Glomerulonephritis, which develops ultimately to uremia and terminal renal failure.

Orally the disease usually starts with tumor like vegetations in mouth and nose (Fig. 22.21). Inflammatory process starts in the interdental papilla, spreading rapidly in to the periodontium. The lesion undergoes necrosis with formation of large perforating ulceration. Involvement of gingiva is the most common manifestation; which is

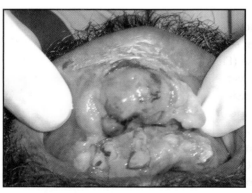

Fig. 22.21: Tumor like vegetation seen in the midline of patient in Wegner's granulomatosis

characterized by ulceration, friable granular lesions or simple enlargement of gingiva. Inflamed, hyperplastic appearing and hemorrhagic gingiva may be found. There may be perforation of palate. There may be loosening of teeth, spontaneous exfoliation of teeth, diffuse ulcerative stomatitis, post-extraction poor healing, cranial nerve palsies and parotid swelling.

Combination of trimethoprim and sulfamethoxazole has proved to be effective as an adjuvant or sole therapy in both localized and generalized forms.

Midline Lethal Granuloma

It is also called as 'malignant granuloma', 'midline lethal granulomatous ulceration' and 'midline non-healing granuloma'. It is described as idiopathic progressive destruction of nose, palate, face and pharynx.

It begins as superficial ulceration of the palate (Fig. 22.22) or nasal septum, often preceded by a feeling of stuffiness in the nose (Fig. 22.22). This may persist for a month or two to several years. Eventually ulceration spreads from the palate to the inside of the nose and then to the outside. The palatal, nasal and malar bones may become involved, undergo necrosis and eventually sequestrate. Destruction is a prominent feature and loss of entire palate is common. The patient may exhibit purulent discharge from the eyes and nose; perforating sinus tracts may develop and soft tissues of face may slough away leaving a direct opening into the nasopharynx and oral cavity.

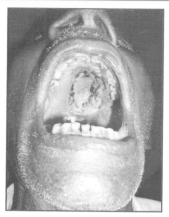

Fig. 22.22: Midline lethal granuloma showing
perforation and ulceration in the palate

Corticosteroid therapy has proven beneficial in some cases. Radiation therapy of 5000 rad appears to be a treatment modality, in which remission of over 15 years is reported.

Disease of Bone Manifested in Jaw

Fibrous Dysplasia

It arises from the bone forming mesenchyme in the spongiosa and develops by proliferation of fibrous tissue. Lichtenstein in 1938 coined the term 'fibrous dysplasia'.

It can be monostotic fibrous dysplasia, polyostotic fibrous dysplasia (Jaffe type and Albright's syndrome).

The skin lesions consist of irregularly pigmented, light brown melanotic spots, described as 'cafe-au-lait spot'. Recurrent bone pain is the most common presenting skeletal symptom. Skeletal lesions may be unilateral in distribution or may involve nearly all bones of the body. Spontaneous fracture is a common complication. In rare cases, continuous and inexorable extension results in great deformity and blindness. Albright's syndrome, in addition show, endocrinal disturbances like precocious puberty, goiter, hyperthyroidism, hyperparathyroidism, Cushing's syndrome and acromegaly.

Orally there may be unilateral facial swelling, which is slow growing with intact overlying mucosa (Fig. 23.1). Swelling is usually painless but patients may feel discomfort

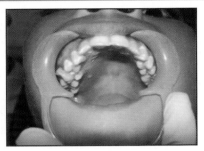

Fig. 23.1: Fibrous dysplasia involving maxillary sinus presented as swelling on the right side

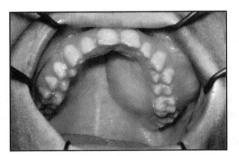

Fig. 23.2: Fibrous dysplasia presented as expansion in the right maxillary area

in some cases and while others complain of frank pain. There is enlarging deformities of alveolar process mainly buccal and labial cortical plates (Fig. 23.2). In mandible, it causes protuberant excrescence of the inferior border of mandible. The teeth present in the affected area are either

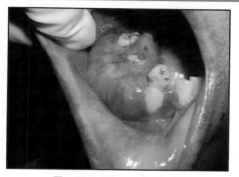

Fig. 23.3: Fibrous dysplasia
(*Courtesy:* Dr Amit Parate, GDCH, Nagpur, India)

malaligned and tipped or displaced (Fig. 23.3). Dental anomalies such as super-numerary teeth have been reported in connection with the monostotic fibrous dysplasia. The most commonly affected site is maxillary midline and mandibular premolar region. These supernumerary teeth often remain impacted and may affect the eruption of normal teeth.

Radiologically it can be radiolucent, mixed or radiopaque depending upon the stage. In early stage there is radiolucency with ill defined borders. Margins may be well defined with a tendency to blend imperceptibly with surrounding normal bone. When the lesion involves the apices of teeth there is loss of lamina dura. Resorption of roots and destruction of developing teeth. In mixed stage radiographic appearance of lesions with heterogeneous distribution of fibrous and osseous tissue show a mixed

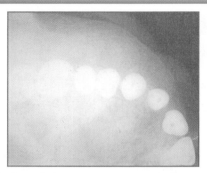

Fig. 23.4: Ground glass appearance seen in fibrous dysplasia

radiolucent and radiopaque appearance, depending on the maturity of the lesions.

In mature stage, the radiograph shows bone of increased density. The normal structure of bone is replaced by a stippled appearance which resembles the ring of orange which is called as 'orange peel'. When mandible is affected, the vertical depth of mandible is increased. The appearance resembles a 'thumb print', as if the bone had been soft and pressed upon by the thumb (Fig. 23.5). Bony expansion usually extends to the buccal and distal aspect. Another characteristic appearance of fibrous dysplasia is ground glass appearance, (Fig. 23.4) also termed as granular. Apart from the appearance everything else is similar as in stippled type.

It is managed by osseous contouring which is necessary for correcting the deformity for esthetics or pre-esthetic purposes.

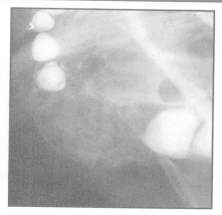

Fig. 23.5: Fibrous dysplasia showing
expansion giving thumb print appearance

Cherubism

It is also known as 'familial fibrous dysplasia of the jaws', 'disseminated juvenile fibrous dysplasia', 'familial multilocular cystic disease of the jaws' and 'hereditary fibrous dysplasia of the jaws'. The clinical entity was first described by Jones in 1933 who coined the term 'Cherubism' reflecting the characteristic chubby facial appearance of affected children.

In the rapidly increasing stage, the child assumes a chubby, cherubic facial appearance, (Fig. 23.6) especially if combined with involvement of the orbital floor with upward displacement of the globe and exposure of the scleral rims.

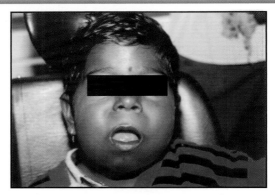

Fig. 23.6: Chubby face appearance seen in Cherubism

The patient may have difficulty in speech, deglutition, mastication, respiration and limited jaw movement (Fig. 23.7). Bilateral enlargement of mandible in this condition produces full, round lower face (Fig. 23.8). Bilateral enlargement of maxilla gradually follows. Pulling or stretching of skin of the cheek, depresses the lower eyelid, exposing a thin line of sclera and resulting in the so called "eyes raised to heaven" look. Swelling is firm and hard on palpation. Overlying mucosa is intact and non-painful.

The fibrous replacement of bone displaces the deciduous dentition. The primary teeth may be irregularly spaced and some may be absent. There is premature loss of primary teeth. The developing permanent teeth are affected, giving rise to displaced unerupted or absent teeth along with malocclusion.

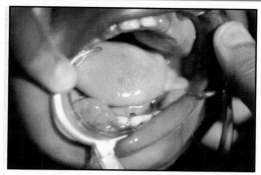

Fig. 23.7: Intraoral swelling seen in patient of cherubism

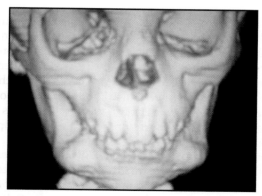

Fig. 23.8: Cherubism showing expansile pattern on both side of the mandible (*Courtesy:* Dr Eswar, Professor and Head, Oral Medicine and Radiology, Sri Ramakrishna Dental College and Hospital, Coimbatore India)

Cyst like radiolucency of mandible, bilaterally symmetrical which is up to several centimeters in diameter. Initiation of bone destruction near the angle of the mandible with later expansion of lesions posteriorly into ramus and anteriorly, into the mandibular body (Fig. 23.8). It appears as a classic multilocular cavity due to internal radiopaque septa, which tends to coalesce as they enlarge. On posteroanterior views, teeth seen to hanging in air. They are well defined, well corticated and smooth around most of the radiolucency. There is also expansion of buccal and lingual cortical plates.

Surgical procedures should be delayed, as long as possible, as the cystic lesion defect usually becomes static and regresses during adulthood.

Central Giant Cell Granuloma

It is a non-neoplastic bone disease reactive to some unknown stimulus. It was first described in the jaws by Waren 1837. It has been called as osteoclastoma, myeloid sarcoma, chronic hemorrhagic osteomyelitis and giant cell reparative granuloma.

The earliest sign of the lesion may be expansion of bone with premature loosening and shedding of deciduous teeth. There is jaw swelling associated with facial asymmetry. Usually painless, but local discomfort may be noted. Palpation may elicit tenderness. Growth is slow. Teeth in the area may become mobile but maintain their vitality, until they are exfoliated.

Radiologically solitary unilocular or multilocular radiolucency. It may occupy whole of the mandibular body

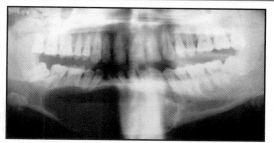

Fig. 23.9: Central giant cell granuloma showing radiolucency which is crossing the midline

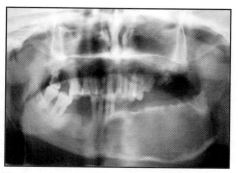

Fig. 23.10: Central giant cell granuloma radiolucency surrounded by well defined margin and crossing the midline

and may extend past the midline to the opposite side (Fig. 23.9). As it grows, it causes bossing of buccal cortex, i.e. uneven, variable bulging or undulation of the cortical contour. Borders may be smooth, undulating, moderately well defined (Fig. 23.10) and moderately well corticated. It shows bony trabeculation within their contour and tends to be mildly wavy on close inspection. Displacement of adjacent teeth, tooth buds and resorption may occur.

It is managed by surgical excision and enucleation.

Paget's Disease

It is also called as 'osteitis deformans'. It was discovered in 1877 by Sir James Paget. There is abnormal resorption and apposition of bone in one or more bones.

First complains may be that patient needs to buy a hat of larger size because of skull enlargement. Bone pain is a consistent symptom and most often directed toward weight bearing areas. Deafness due to involvement of the petrous portion of temporal bone with compression of cochlear nerve in the foramen. Mental disturbance, dizziness. Bowing of legs, curvature of spine and enlargement of skull. The involved bones are warm to touch because of increased vascularity and are prone to fracture. Broadening and flattening of the chest and spinal curvature. The patient assumes Waddling gait.

Orally movement and migration of affected teeth, malocclusion and in edentulous patient poor fit of denture. Increase in alveolar width associated (Fig. 23.11) with flattening of palate when maxilla is involved. As the disease progresses the mouth may remain open exposing the teeth as the lips are too small to cover the enlarged jaws. Extraction sites heal slowly and incidences of osteomyelitis are higher.

Radiologically it appearance as early radiolucent stage (Inferior cortex may appear osteoporotic and possess a

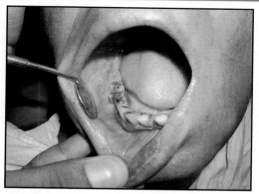

Fig. 23.11: Paget's disease showing widened ridge

laminated structure. Bone pattern in which trabeculae though reduced in number, run linearly in the direction of length of bone and have few inter-sections between them. Root resorption is common. In the skull, early lytic lesion may be seen as discrete radiolucent areas termed as osteoporosis circumscripta), granular or ground glass appearance (there are rounded radiopaque patches of abnormal bone of greater density within the radiolucent bone, within which it is not possible to see any actual bone structure), a dense , more radiopaque stage (In later stages, rounded radiopaque patches of abnormal bone are often seen giving an impression of cotton wool. As the fully opacified area becomes more numerous and enlarged, they tend to coalesce). Hypercementosis may be produced on one or more teeth (Fig. 23.12). It may obliterate areas of

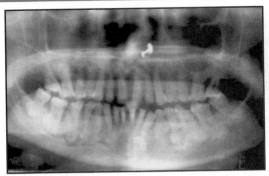

Fig. 23.12: Generalized hypercementosis seen in case of Paget's disease (*Courtesy:* Dr Chandrashekhar Bande, Lecturer, Oral Surgery, GDCH, Nagpur, India)

lamina dura and periodontal ligament space around both, normal and hypercementosed roots resulting in ankylosis of teeth.

It is managed by calcitonin, a parathyroid hormone antagonist produced by the thyroid gland, suppresses bone resorption and also relieves pain and decrease serum alkaline. Another option available are surgery and radiation therapy.

Florid Osseous Dysplasia

It is also called as 'gigantiform cementoma', 'chronic sclerosing osteomyelitis', 'sclerosing osteitis', 'multiple enostosis' and 'sclerotic cemental masses'. It is considered to be a widespread form of periapical dysplasia. It is derived from the cells in or near the periodontal ligament space.

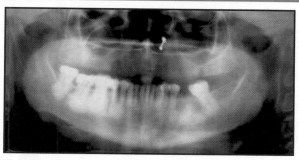

Fig. 23.13: Florid osseous dysplasia involving most the mandibular region with oval radiopacity (*Courtesy:* Dr Amit Parate, Lecturer, Oral Medicine and Radiology, GDCH, Nagpur, India)

There is a painless expansion of the alveolar process of mandible. Patients may complain of intermittent poorly localized pain in the affected bone area, with or without an associated bony swelling. Mucosal ulceration with fistulous tract may be present. Teeth are vital.

Radiologically there is radiolucent cavity, partially filled with one or more dense radiopaque masses. As lesions mature, the radiopacities increase (Fig. 23.13). The overall appearance is that of an amorphous mixed radiolucent and radiopaque lesion. Lobular or lump shaped and soft radiopaque characters like that of cotton wool. Margins are fairly regular and well defined. Each lesion is surrounded by a radiolucent capsule and a cortical rim. It involves all four quadrants. Hypercementosis of tooth in the affected area is seen.

If teeth present effective oral hygiene should be maintained since with this disease, patients exhibit poor healing and osteomyelitis may develop after tooth loss.

Ossifying Fibroma

It is characteristically encapsulated neoplasm consisting of highly cellular fibrous tissue in which bone formation occurs. They may show a locally aggressive behavior.

Occasional facial asymmetry is seen in some of the cases. When in maxilla, symptoms may include nasal stuffiness and epiphora on the affected side. There may be associated exophthalmos, with visual disturbances, depending on the extent of compression of its orbital content by the tumor. The lesion is slow growing and in some cases, there is displacement of teeth. Bony cortex and covering mucosa remain intact. The lesion may be slow growing initially, with a rapid increase in size in a relatively short time (Fig. 23.14). If sinus is affected it may fill the sinus completely and expands the sinus wall.

Radiologically bone destruction occurs early in the tumor formation, represented by radiolucent defect within the bone. Bone destruction enlarge concentrically. There is tendency of bone destruction occurring beneath the periosteum. Subsequent calcification results in the appearance of radiopaque foci. The radiopaque calcified masses tend to coalesce and tumor may become radiopaque after some years. Borders are well defined with thin radiolucent lines representing the fibrous capsule separating the lesion.

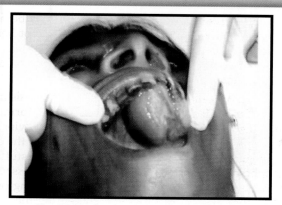

Fig. 23.14: Giant ossifying fibroma involving
maxillary upper left region

Conservatively enucleated and the tissue is examined microscopically to establish the final diagnosis.

Osteoporosis

There is reduction in the inorganic constituent. There is abnormal persistence of calcified cartilage. Spongy portion of affected bone ultimately becomes a solid block of calcified cartilage leaving inadequate space for hemopoiesis.

Bones are fragile and susceptible to fracture. Osteoporotic patient may notice gradual loss of height due to shortening of trunk. In advanced cases clinical onset is often characterized by attack of severe pain which is aggravated by movements and occurs after trauma.

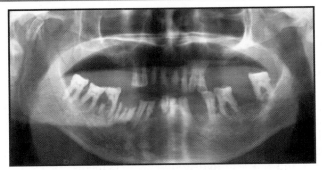

Fig. 23.15: Osteoporosis
(*Courtesy:* Dr Amit Parate, GDCH, Nagpur, India)

Orally there may be fracture of jaws during tooth extraction. Enamel hypoplasia. Microscopic dentinal defect. Arrested root development, retardation of tooth eruption. Delayed eruption and early loss of teeth missing teeth and malformed teeth.

Radiologically typical wedge appearance of affected vertebrae occurs on a lateral radiograph. Reduction in number of trabeculae is least evident in the alveolar process. Persistent trabeculae tend to occur along planes of bone stress. Trabeculae may be arranged in a radial manner, with wide spaces in between. Reduced density and thinning of cortical boundaries, such as inferior mandibular cortex (Fig. 23.15). The lamina dura surrounding the teeth may appear thinner than normal.

Good nutrition and regular exercise helps to prevent osteoporosis.

Osteopetrosis

It is also called as 'Marble bone disease', 'Albers-Schonberg disease', 'osteosclerosis fragilis generalisata'. It is a rare disorder characterized by an increase in density of bones, which becomes hard and brittle.

As a result of continuous bone deposition and lack of bone resorption, the foramina of cranial nerves are constricted, hence there is loss of hearing, disturbed vision, which diminish progressively. Facial nerve palsy is also seen. There is also frontal bossing, obliteration of maxillary sinus and possible hydrocephalus and mental retardation.

Orally osteomyelitis of jaws associated with osteo-petrosis probably follows the obliteration and fibrosis of marrow is caused by reduced osseous circulation. Paranasal sinus may become readily obliterated.

Radiologically there is diffuse homogeneous sclerotic appearance of all bones, within distinction between the cortex and the marrow (Fig. 23.16). The changes in the skull are often striking. The base of skull becomes grossly thickened and of great radiographic density. Loss of normal skull marking and structures. Due to increased calcification there is increased fragility, so fractures are common. Less marked changes may produce increase in overall density but trabeculation may be apparent (Fig. 23.17). The trabeculae may get thickened and the marrow spaces are correspondingly small (Fig. 23.16). The lamina dura is almost lost in the general density.

Avoid major surgery in patients with osteopetrosis. Performing dental extraction has a risk of osteomyelitis and jaw fracture.

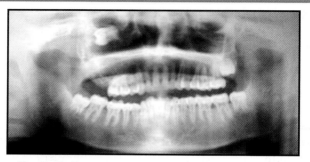

Fig. 23.16: Osteopetrosis of the jaw (*Courtesy:* Dr Datarkar, Associate Professor, Oral Surgery, SPDC Wardha, India)

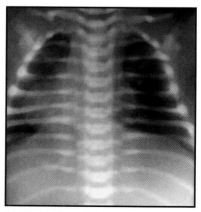

Fig. 23.17: Marble bone disease showing sclerotic appearance of bone (*Courtesy:* Dr A K Ganju, Clinical Hematologist, Nagpur, India)

Osteogenesis Imperfecta

It is also called as 'brittle bone', 'Lobstein disease'. It is a serious disease of unknown etiology. It represents a hereditary autosomal dominant trait.

Extreme fragility and porosity of bones with an attendant proneness of fracture. Fracture heals readily but new bone is of similar imperfection. It is common for fracture to occur while the infant is walking or crawling. Hyperplastic callus formations, which may mimic osteosarcoma, take place (Fig. 23.18). There is occurrence of pale blue sclera which is

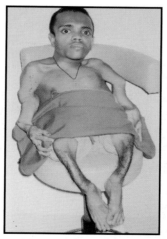

Fig. 23.18: Osteogenesis imperfecta showing deformity (*Courtesy:* Dr MN Naidu, Dr Pravin Lambade, Oral and Maxillofacial Surgery, CDCRI, Rajnandgao, India)

thin; pigmented choroid shows through and produces the blue color. There is deafness due to osteosclerosis; laxity of ligament and peculiar shape of the skull (Fig. 23.18). There is also abnormal electrical reaction of muscle. Increased tendency for capillary bleeding.

Orally there is hypoplasia of teeth. Some time there is class I malocclusion and grater incidence of impacted 1st and 2nd molars. Deciduous teeth are poorly calcified and semi-translucent or waxy. Appearance of teeth is faint dirty pink, half normal size, with globular crowns and relatively short roots in proportion to other dimension.

Radiologically patient may show wormian bone (bones in skull sutures) (Fig. 23.19), skeletal deformities and

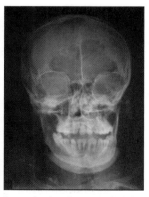

Fig. 23.19: Skull radiograph showing wormian bone (*Courtesy:* Dr MN Naidu, Dr Pravin Lambade, Oral and Maxillofacial Surgery, CDCRI, Rajnandgao, India)

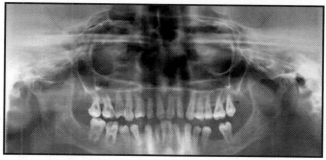

Fig. 23.20: Osteoporotic bone seen in case of osteogenesis imperfecta (*Courtesy:* Dr MN Naidu, Dr Pravin Lambade, Oral and Maxillofacial surgery, CDCRI, Rajnandgao, India)

progressive osteopenia. The bone is osteoporotic, there is less density and trabeculae are fewer in number (Fig. 23.20). The chin is sharply pointed, as a result of softening of bone, leading to flattening of sides of the mandible.

No known treatment.

Massive Osteolysis

It is also called as 'vanishing bone', 'disappearing bone', 'phantom bone', 'progressive osteolysis or 'Gorham syndrome'. It is characterized by spontaneous, progressive resorption of bone with ultimate total disappearance of bone.

The disease may or may not be painful, begins suddenly and advance rapidly, until the involved bone is replaced by a thin layer of fibrous tissue surrounding a cavity.

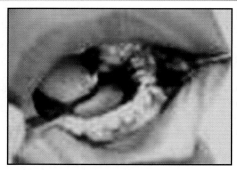

Fig. 23.21: Intraoral features of vanishing bone disease (*Courtesy:* Dr Chandrashekhar Kadam, Lecturer, Rangoonwala Dental College, Pune)

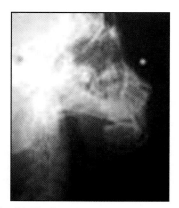

Fig. 23.22: Complete destruction of bone occur in massive osteolysis

Orally the patients may present with pain or facial asymmetry, (Fig. 23.21) or both and there is pathologic fracture of bone following even minor trauma. There may be complete destruction of mandible; maxilla is less commonly affected.

Radiologically there is complete destruction of bone occur (Fig. 23.22).

There is no specific treatment; although surgical resection ceases the progress of the disease.

Index